Childhood
Ear Infections

The Family Health Series

Childhood Ear Infections

What Every Parent and Physician Should Know About Prevention, Home Care, and Alternative Treatment

by
Dr. Michael A. Schmidt

Foreword by
Lendon H. Smith, Pediatrician
and Author of *Feed Your Kids Right*

North Atlantic Books
Homeopathic Educational Services
Berkeley, California

Childhood Ear Infections:
What Every Parent and Physician Should Know
About Prevention, Home Care, and Alternative Treatment

Publishers' Addresses:

North Atlantic Books	Homeopathic Educational Services
P.O. Box 12327	2124 Kittredge Street
Berkeley, California 94701	Berkeley, California 94704

Cover and book design by Paula Morrison
Photo of Zoltan von Bozzay by George Fuller-von Bozzay
Typeset by Campaigne & Associates Typography

Childhood Ear Infections is sponsored by The Society for the Study of Native Arts and Sciences, a nonprofit educational corporation whose goals are to develop an educational and crosscultural perspective linking various scientific, social and artistic fields; to nurture a holistic view of arts, sciences, humanities, and healing; and to publish and distribute literature on the relationship of mind, body and nature.

This book discusses the problem of childhood ear infections. It has been written as an educational guide and reference for both laypersons and health care professionals, but it is not intended to replace the services of a physician. Treatment of any illness must be supervised by a licensed health care professional. The author and publisher disclaim all responsibility arising from any adverse effects or results that might occur as a result of the application of any of the information contained in this book. Accordingly, either your or the professional who examines and treats you must take full responsibility for the uses made of this book. Before undertaking any of the self-care treatments described in this book it is advisable to consult your health care professional.

Library of Congress Cataloging-in-Publication Data

Schmidt, Michael A., 1958–
    Childhood ear infections: what every parent and physician should know about prevention, home cure and alternative treatment/Michael A. Schmidt.
        p.   cm.—(The family health series)
    Includes bibliographical references and index.
    ISBN 1–55643–089–2 (paper)   ISBN 1–55643–102–3 (cloth)
    1. Otitis media in children.   I. Title.   II. Series.
RF225.S36   1990
618.92'09784—dc20   90–7868
                                                                  CIP

To my wife Julie and my son Caleb.

Acknowledgments

I am grateful:

To the editors of the *Journal of Chinese Medicine* and Dr. Julian Scott for granting me liberal use of their material on pediatric acupuncture.

To Dr. Martha Benedict for her time and valuable insights into the management of otitis media. To Anastacia White, a professional herbalist specializing in Chinese botanical medicine. Her contribution to the chapter on botanical medicine was invaluable. To Dr. Stephen Messer for the use of his graphics on homeopathic medicine.

To computer programmer Michael Koenigs, who saved this manuscript after my computer suffered a near disastrous system crash. Without his efforts, this book would probably not exist.

To the late Dr. Robert S. Mendelsohn, a champion of children and opponent of the overuse of medical procedures. He is sorely missed by all of us who knew and loved him as a gentle man and brilliant doctor. I will miss his wit, determination, and relentless pursuit of simplicity and wholism in the rapidly changing world of medicine.

To John Harder of Duluth, Minnesota for his excellent illustrations. To the numerous others who played small but important roles in the evolution of this book: Dr. Susan Esch, Steven Gresham, Frank and Janice Moinicken, Dr. Paul Westby, Greg Peterson, Carl Neubauer, and Dr. Lendon H. Smith.

To my patients—both children and adults—who challenged me to be a good diagnostician, a compassionate listener, and to learn more.

To the staff at the University of Minnesota Biomedical Information Services and to Marcia Stevens at Northwestern College of Chiropractic for their assistance in searching the medical literature. To the many doctors who have performed the rigorous research referenced in this book.

To my editor Dana Ullman, whose constructive ideas and thoughtful insights helped mold this book into its present shape. To Richard Grossinger for his help in guiding this book to publication. To Kathy Glass for helping to give this book clarity and consistency.

To my parents, El and Dorothy Schmidt, who throughout my life have been supportive of all that I've done.

A special thanks to my wife Julie, who endured long hours of editing and my ceaseless absence while I worked on this project. It is her love, support, and understanding that has given me the privilege to write.

Above all, I thank God for giving me the talent, energy, and opportunity to share my ideas and contribute to the welfare of children through this book.

Contents

Figures

Foreword

A Letter from Dr. Lendon H. Smith to Dr. Michael A. Schmidt

As a pediatrician I *knew* how to treat otitis media: give the child penicillin, sulfa drug, or ampicillin and take another look in 10 days. If it is all cleared up, fine. If not, send the child to an ENT specialist for myringotomy and adenoidectomy. But why did they get sick in the first place? Their parents loved them, wanted them, fed them well, and even gave vitamins. I was confused when parents would ask, "Why is he sick all the time?" We never got a course about *reasons* in our medical training. It was just make a diagnosis and write out the prescription. The pharmaceutical companies told us that we should become good diagnosticians; they would provide the treatment protocol.

You have brought up some embarrassing questions and also have made some connections about which we had no knowledge. But you are right. There are reasons for everything.

You have given us the reasons, and some new ways of looking at some old problems. In a clear and logical fashion you have outlined the factors involved in—not just ear infections—but sickness in general. Your revelation of the connection between fats and infection-susceptibility is a classic; I have never read anything so easy to understand. The chapter on alternative treatment is especially valuable because it shows parents that methods other than antibtiotics and surgery are being used to care for earaches. This chapter is valuable to doctors because it outlines the details of these methods.

You have thoroughly researched the field and have carefully separated out the logical from the spurious. You are careful to state if you have found some real controversy in the treatment of otitis media. The general public should have your book as a ready reference so that the average parent can confront the treating doctor with the published studies.

xiii

Not every red ear needs to be treated. I am aware now that when I gave a shot of some antibiotic to a child, the child got better—but often from the "tincture of time" rather than the therapy itself. How easily we can delude ourselves. I remember a house call I made on a feverish one-year-old child. The eardrums were red, but there was no bulging or evidence of pus. I gave a shot of penicillin anyway, because I thought I ought to be doing something. Within a day or two the fever dropped to normal and the next day the child developed a measle-like rash all over his trunk. It was roseola, baby measles. The mother is still convinced the child is allergic to penicillin.

Dr. Schmidt, you have done a great service to the sick children and the worried parents of the world, and, I hope, to the pediatricians and otolaryngologists who should know better.

Dr. Lendon H. Smith
Pediatrician and author
of *Feed Your Kids Right*

Introduction

Ear infections are the number-one reason parents bring their children to the doctor. Over the last ten years, the number of children who get earaches has risen sharply. As a parent and a doctor, I am concerned about the high numbers of children affected by this illness and about what conventional medicine has to offer. Certainly, we all know there are children with ear infections who have been benefited by antibiotics and tubes. But, we also know those who have not been helped. Indeed, there are even children who have been hurt by these forms of treatment.

Because of this, I have spent considerable time investigating the current medical methods of treatment and the alternatives that are available. One would not know from the popular press that doctors are not wholly successful at treating ear infections in children. It is surprising that the media has not addressed this. But there is now evidence that demands we take a new look at an old and growing problem. Consider these findings:

- When antibiotics are used at the beginning of an acute middle ear infection, the frequency of recurrent infections may be almost three times greater than if antibiotics are delayed or not used.[1]

- Antibiotics have been shown not to affect the outcome of acute middle ear infection with regard to pain, fever, hearing, and healing time.[2]

- There appears to be little difference in outcome of middle ear infections treated with a three-day course of antibiotic when compared with those treated with the typical ten-day course of antibiotic.[3]

- Eardrum scarring with membrane thickening has been found to occur in over 40 percent of children receiving tubes compared with zero percent in those not receiving tubes.[4]

- Many cases of chronic middle ear infection, even those with eardrum perforation, are due to allergy.[5]

- In up to 70 percent of children with middle ear "infection" who do not respond to antibiotics, the middle ear fluid contains *no* harmful bacteria.[6]

- Zinc deficient children suffer from more ear infections than those with normal zinc status. There is evidence that nutrition may play a crucial role in the prevention and treatment of recurrent ear infections.[7]

In this book, I examine the scope of the ear infection problem. I take a careful look at the current methods of treatment. Antibiotics and tubes are discussed in depth because they are the most frequently used methods of treatment. They are not, however, without risk or side effect. I take a new look at causes of ear infections and present a discussion of diet and nutrition that has significant implications. The home care and prevention chapters are valuable to parents because of the practical information they contain. What may ultimately be most useful is the section on alternative treatment, in which I describe the methods used by holistic doctors to treat earaches.

My purpose is not to condemn conventional medicine, since I recognize its inherent value and tremendous contributions. However, we must realize that medicine is a collaborative effort—one that embraces the useful features of all healing systems. It is my hope that the medicine of the twenty-first century will be a mixture of the science of medicine and the art of healing, that it will be a way of viewing the patient as a whole, while understanding the function of his parts. It is only after such a synthesis that we can say our system of healing has evolved to truly serve the needs of our children and ourselves.

Dr. Michael A. Schmidt
April, 1990

Chapter I

The Scope
of the Problem

*"The treatment of recurrent otitis media remains an unre-
solved problem."* [1]

Leon Eisenberg, M.D.

Tiffany was just nine months old when she experienced her
first ear infection. It began with sleepless nights, irritability,
and fussiness at dinner time. Before long it was obvious that
she was ill and needed attention. Her parents took her to the
pediatrician. Diagnosis—acute otitis media. Tiffany was treated
with antibiotics. Within two weeks, her ears improved, but
within four weeks, the ear infection had returned.

Back to the pediatrician. Tiffany's doctor again prescribed
antibiotics. After two weeks, she showed improvement. But
the ear infection returned within four weeks. The cycle continued. By the time Tiffany was twenty-one months old, she
had received antibiotics on eleven separate occasions—all to
no avail. Tiffany's parents were exhausted and frustrated. They
felt helpless at their inability to do anything for their daughter.
The effects of repeated antibiotics concerned them. When Tiffany was two and a half years old, her parents agreed to have
tubes put in her ears.

The tubes seemed to help. At the beginning, Tiffany could
hear somewhat better and the earaches subsided. Gradually,
fluid returned and hearing started to diminish. Tiffany was
weak, sickly, and irritable. The cycle was starting again.

Ear infections . . . antibiotics . . . more ear infections . . . more antibiotics . . . ear infections . . . antibiotics. This is the recurring theme for millions of infants and toddlers each year. For many children with recurrent earaches, tubes are the ultimate fate. Yet, in spite of repeated antibiotics and tubes, many children continue to have problems until they are six or seven years old—an age when earaches subside naturally. Tiffany was headed in this direction, but her parents chose a different course.

When Tiffany was four, her parents had grown weary of the unsuccessful attempts to cure her earaches. On the recommendation of a friend, Tiffany's parents took her to a doctor who used natural methods to care for earaches. The new doctor explained that Tiffany had dietary and nutritional problems that previous doctors had not addressed. Tiffany was placed on a diet free of dairy products, eggs, and sulfites—foods to which she tested sensitive. The doctor also prescribed specific nutrients and homeopathic medicines. Within one month of beginning this program, her middle ear effusion cleared. Within two months, her ears had recovered fully. Today Tiffany is eleven years old. The ear infection she had at age four was her last. She has completely recovered from the hearing problems she suffered as a small child and is on the A honor roll at school. (See chapter 6 for additional details about Tiffany's tubes.)

Tiffany's recovery was swift. Not all ear infections managed in this way improve so quickly. But this case illustrates the value of using natural forms of healing for childhood illness. Tiffany's case is just one of many cases of childhood ear infections treated successfully by doctors around the world using natural methods.

In this book, we'll explore a variety of natural healing methods that are used to care for earaches, along with valuable tips about prevention and home care. Before moving on to this discussion, it is important that you understand some basic things about childhood ear infections—what they are, how they're treated, who's at risk, and complications.

Otitis media, or middle ear inflammation, is the number-one childhood health problem in America. In one survey, it was found to be the most frequently diagnosed illness and the most frequent reason, after well-baby and child care, for visits to a doctor.[2] The diagnosis and treatment of middle ear problems accounts for roughly one-third of all pediatric visits,[3] comprising roughly 30 million visits to the doctor per year.[4] The overall cost of diagnosis and treatment now exceeds 2.2 billion dollars annually.[5]

For many children, earaches begin in infancy. By the age of three, over two-thirds of all children have had one or more episodes of acute otitis media, including 33 percent who have had three or more episodes.[6] Nearly all children affected continue to have problems until the age of six or seven. Otitis media does not become rare until after age 10,[7] and persists in some children beyond 15 years of age. Boys appear to be affected more often than girls in the younger age groups, while the trend reverses in older children.[8]

In spite of vast increases in the pediatric use of antibiotics, the incidence of otitis media has risen sharply. Most recent evidence shows that from 1977 to 1986, office visits for otitis media have soared by 136 percent.[9] This substantial increase in otitis media has been attributed to everything from increased doctor awareness to improved diagnostic abilities. There are even those who contend that the incidence of otitis media has increased, in part, *because* of the widespread use of antibiotic drugs.[10] To a degree, any of the above explanations may have merit. However, there are additional factors that have emerged during the past several decades that increase a child's susceptibility to illness such as otitis media. These will be explored in later chapters.

What is an Earache?

An earache can develop when the tissue lining the middle ear or eustachian tube swells (See figure 1-a.). As the membranes

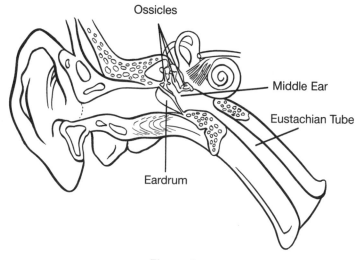

Figure 1-a
Structures of the Ear

swell, the opening of the eustachian tube gradually becomes obstructed, thereby preventing the middle ear from draining properly. As inflammation of the middle ear builds, the production of fluid increases. In some cases bacteria contribute to the ongoing inflammation, while in others the inflammatory response occurs for different reasons.

The congestion within the middle ear causes pressure to be exerted on the eardrum and the sensitive structures that lie within (and near) the middle ear chamber. The pressure exerted on the eardrum can produce one of the most painful sensations your child will ever experience. When the eustachian tube is blocked, there is no way to alter the pressure in the middle ear. In some cases, the eardrum ruptures and fluid drains out, which reduces the pressure. In others, the inflammation subsides and the eustachian tube opens, allowing drainage of fluid. Sometimes treatment is required to encourage proper function of the eustachian tube and reduced production of fluid in the middle ear.

Signs and Symptoms

It may be surprising to know that many instances of otitis media occur with a relative absence of symptoms. Your child may act and hear normally and experience no pain. Yet if the doctor examined the eardrum during a routine physical or for another reason, he may see fluid behind the eardrum. Fluid may even drain from the ear with no other evidence that the child is having problems. Chronic ear infections often occur with little pain. Acute ear infections can be severely painful. In general, pain is one of the most common signs of middle ear problems.

One of the first indicators of a middle ear problem is a change in behavior or sleep habits. This is not specific, however, and could suggest any number of other problems. A child may pull or tug at the ear or frequently poke his finger into the ear canal. This also might indicate itchiness in the ear or a foreign object lodged in the canal. An abrupt or temporary change in hearing acuity may signal a middle ear problem as well.

Older children who can better communicate their feelings might complain of a plugged, blocked, or pressure sensation in the middle ear. Buzzing or ringing sensations may occur.

Symptoms of acute earaches commonly include (although all may not be present in a given child):

- Ear pain.
- Fever.
- Drainage from the ear.
- Sleeplessness.
- Irritability.
- Change in eating habits.
- Change in hearing.
- Refusal to nurse on one side.
- Nasal obstruction or discharge.

In cases of chronic earache, the most notable symptom might be diminished hearing. Behavior changes are also common.

How the Doctor Diagnoses an Ear Infection

The most common method used by all doctors is visual inspection of the eardrum using an otoscope. The otoscope is the familiar hand-held device you've seen the doctor use when looking in your child's ears. When looking in the ear, the appearance of the eardrum is the most important sign. The eardrum has several characteristic landmarks. If any of these landmarks have changed in appearance, it may suggest a problem in the middle ear.

Since the eardrum is somewhat transparent, it is possible to see behind it to a limited degree. Behind the eardrum the doctor might observe an arrangement of large or small bubbles—suggesting fluid in the middle ear—or a fluid line. This fluid line will often change position when the child tips her head forward or backward (just as if you had taken a glass full of water and tipped it back and forth).

The eardrum is normally pearly-grey and shiny. If it loses its luster, problems may be present. Redness of the eardrum or the ear canal is one of the first signs for which a doctor looks. However, redness of the eardrum is not a reliable basis for diagnosing a middle ear infection.[11] Redness can occur because of allergy, high fever, inflammation or infection. Crying, which is typical of a sick child undergoing a middle ear exam, can lead to a temporary engorgement of the blood vessels in the ear canal and also can give a bright red appearance to the eardrum. This should not be mistaken for an ear infection.

A variation of the otoscope is the pneumatic otoscope. This device is an otoscope that has been modified by attaching a tube that connects to a small bulb. In an examination, the doctor places the speculum in the ear as usual. A tight seal of the speculum against the ear canal is needed so that no air escapes. The doctor then pumps air into the external ear chamber using the bulb. Pumping air into this sealed chamber causes the normal eardrum to be forced away from the doctor. When the air pressure is released, the eardrum returns to its normal position. If the middle ear is full of fluid or pus, the eardrum moves very little or not at all. When done properly, pneumatic otoscopy is a very useful way to find out if there is fluid in the middle ear.

Tympanometry is another method used to examine for middle ear effusion or fluid. Like the pneumatic otoscope, the tympanometer uses air pumped into the ear canal to assess movement of the eardrum. The major difference is that as air is drawn out of the ear canal, a sonic signal is bounced off the eardrum. As the air is gradually released, the response of the eardrum is monitored electronically and plotted on a graph— called a tympanogram. You may have heard your doctor refer to a "flat" tympanogram, meaning that the response of the ear- drum to tympanometry did not produce the typical spiked curve. This suggests there is middle ear fluid. Tympanometry has some drawbacks. It is used more widely in hospitals and large clinics than in small clinics, because of technical consid- erations and cost.

Reflectometry is an accurate and simple method that relies on soundwaves to detect fluid in the middle ear.

All of these methods are used to varying degrees.

Terminology

There are a number of technical terms used throughout this book, and by your doctor, to describe earaches. Some of these may sound confusing. The medical term for problems of the middle ear is **otitis media**, derived from the Latin, oto- mean- ing ear, and -itis meaning inflammation. The term media means middle. Thus, otitis media technically means middle ear inflam- mation—not infection.

Other commonly used terms to describe illness involving the middle ear include:

Chronic and Acute: Refer to duration.
Chronic conditions are those that are recurrent and of long-standing duration. Acute conditions are usually associated with severe symptoms and are of short duration. A child can have chronic otitis media and still suffer from acute episodes.

Serous, Mucoid, and Purulent: Refer to the type of fluid present.
Serous fluid is thin and watery, and usually does not contain harmful bacteria. This type of fluid is very common. Mucoid fluid is thick, sticky, and mucus-like. Purulent (also called suppurative) refers to the presence of fluid that contains many white blood cells—what we typically call pus. This is the type that usually contains harmful bacteria.

Effusion: Refers to the escape of fluid into the middle ear.

Doctors combine the above terms to describe the part involved, the specific region, whether it contains fluid, the type of fluid, and the duration of the problem. For instance, a diagnosis of chronic serous otitis media with effusion implies that there is fluid drainage into the middle ear that is recurring and of long-standing duration.

Throughout this book, I will use the terms earache, otitis media, and ear infection interchangably. I continue to use the term ear infection out of familiarity to the reader. This term is often used inappropriately since not all earaches result from bacterial infection. As we'll see in chapter 5, the middle ear fluid in a high percentage of cases of otitis media contains either *no* bacteria, or *normal* bacteria. In only a small percentage of cases does it contain viruses. Therefore, recognize that not all "ear infections" are actually infections.

Who's at Risk

There are numerous factors that can put your child at increased risk to developing middle ear infection or inflammation. You may be able to reduce your child's chances of developing ear infections by addressing those risk factors that apply to her. Recognize that doctors disagree on the importance of some risk factors.

Season. The incidence of earaches is clearly highest in the winter, with the frequency decreasing in both spring and fall, and declining further in the summer. In northern climates, ear problems become more frequent beginning in September and begin to subside by April.[12]

Cow's Milk Consumption. Early consumption of cow's milk appears to predispose a child to early otitis media. Cow's milk consumption is one of the most significant contributors to middle ear problems in children.[13]

Feeding Position. In one study of more than 2,500 children, the practice of giving a child a bottle in bed was the most important factor associated with persistent fluid in the middle ear.[14] This is, in part, due to the horizontal position of the eustachian tube, and the ease with which fluid backs up into the tube. (See figure 1-b.)

Smoking. Children living in homes where one or more adult smokes develop otitis media at a much higher rate than children living in homes without smokers.[15]

Fetal Alcohol Exposure. A child whose mother has consumed alcohol during gestation is at high risk to developing fetal alcohol syndrome. Otitis media occurs in as many as 93 percent of children with fetal alcohol syndrome.[16]

Figure 1-b
Comparison of the Infant and Adult Eustachian Tube

Genetics. Nearly 60 percent of all children with Down syndrome suffer from otitis media.[17]

Day Care. Children spending time in day care settings have twice the chance of developing otitis media as children minded at home, and are at increased risk to developing illnesses of all types.[18]

Allergy. Many studies show that children with a personal or family history of allergy are more likely to develop otitis media than non-allergic children.[19]

Nutritional Status. Children with deficiency of certain vitamins, minerals, and fatty acids are at risk to developing middle ear problems.[20]

Respiratory Problems. Nearly 50 percent of all cases of otitis media are preceded by an upper respiratory problem of some type (bronchial congestion, nasal congestion, asthma, colds, etc.).[21]

Injury. Children suffering trauma at birth such as that due to forceps, vacuum extraction, or prolonged and difficult labor are at risk to developing otitis media. Included in this category are children who have taken falls and suffered minor injury to the head and neck.[22]

Early Introduction of Solids. Middle ear problems often begin shortly after a baby begins to eat solid foods. The earlier solids are introduced, the greater the likelihood of developing otitis media.

Early Episodes of Otitis Media. Children who experience their first episode of otitis media in the first year of life are more likely to suffer from multiple recurrences of middle ear problems and persistent fluid.[23]

Low Socioeconomic Status. Children living in low socioeconomic conditions are at increased risk to otitis media. They are also at increased risk to those learning problems and developmental delays that are reported to occur in some children with recurrent otitis media.[24]

Current Medical Treatment

The medical treatment of otitis media involves a two-tiered approach consisting of drugs and surgery. Among the drugs used are antibiotics, antihistamines, and decongestants. Antiinflammatory agents are often used to manage fever and pain. The surgical methods include tonsillectomy, adenoidectomy, myringotomy, and tympanostomy. When to use each of these approaches and for what length of time depends largely upon the individual doctor. As one prominent researcher states, "Recommendations regarding the management of secretory otitis

media must be based to a considerable extent on opinion."[25]
   The treatments and a brief note about each are listed below.

Antibiotics

The antibiotics most commonly used in acute otitis media
include penicillin V (first choice in Scandinavian countries),
amoxicillin (first choice in America), other representatives of
the ampicillin group, trimethoprim-sulfmethoxazole, erythro-
mycin combined with a short-acting sulfonamide, and cefaclor.[26]
   The consensus within the medical community is that antibiotics are effective at managing otitis media. However, not
all children respond well to antibiotics, evidenced by the considerable number of children who continue to have middle ear
fluid despite antibiotic therapy. There is evidence that suggests
antibiotics are being overused in the care of earaches. (See
chapter 2.)

Cortisone

Cortisone is not widely used in otitis media. However, because
many earaches are due to inflammation rather than infection,
cortisone continues to be investigated as a therapeutic tool.
Cortisone is used to treat the inflammatory aspects of otitis
media. It works by interfering with the manufacture of a group
of compounds known as inflammatory prostaglandins. (See
chapter 5.)
   Cortisone does not appear to be successful as a sole treatment for otitis media. It has many side effects, and the long-
term impact on the health of children (and indeed the course
of otitis media) is unknown. In one study, its use led to an
increase in middle ear fluid.[27] Recent evidence suggests that
cortisone may interfere with the body's ability to manufacture
its own anti-inflammatory compounds.

Anti-Inflammatory Agents (Aspirin, Tylenol)

Drugs such as aspirin and acetaminophen (found in Tylenol)
are not used as a principal therapy in otitis media, but are used

freely to manage some of the symptoms and discomfort associated with earache including aches, pains, and fever. However, use of these drugs may actually prolong illness and lead to more inflammation. According to Dr. T.T.K. Jung, anti-inflammatory drugs may cause a case of secretory otitis media to degenerate into a case of mucoid otitis media[28] (one that is more resistant to treatment). In other words, if you use aspirin or acetaminophen to make your child more comfortable during an ear infection, there is a chance that the middle ear will get worse and take longer to heal. (See chapter 5.)

This evidence is supported by recent findings reported in the *Journal of Pediatrics*, where acetaminophen (Tylenol) was shown to prolong the course of chicken pox. Many doctors now believe that acetaminophen also may prolong the course of other childhood infections, and that pain and fever reducers such as this should be used sparingly.[29]

Doctors have for some time recommended against giving aspirin to small children during an infection, because of the possibility that aspirin may trigger the development of Reye's syndrome. Reye's syndrome is an often-fatal inflammation of the brain.

Antihistamines/Decongestants

Theoretically, antihistamines should have value in the treatment of otitis media, at least in cases that are believed to be related to allergy. (Antihistamines block the release of histamine, and histamine release by white blood cells is part of the allergic response.) It is also logical that decongestants might work because they dry up the mucous membranes. However, some studies have shown that these drugs are of limited value in treating otitis media. The question seems to have been settled by the results of a study reported in the *New England Journal of Medicine* in 1983. In this double-blind trial, it was shown that children with otitis media who received decongestants and antihistamines fared no better than those who did not. Even allergic children fared no better than non-allergic children.[30]

Tympanostomy

Tympanostomy refers to the placement of tubes in the eardrum. While this procedure is the most common surgery performed on children, many doctors believe it's used too frequently. Recent clinical trials have reported conflicting results regarding the effectiveness of tympanostomy. This is discussed in detail in chapter 3.

Tonsillectomy

The removal of tonsils was once the preferred surgical method of treating otitis media, but has now been replaced by tympanostomy. Swollen tonsils can obstruct the eustachian tube, thereby preventing the middle ear from draining properly. Doctors believe that by removing the tonsils, the eustachian tube opening becomes unblocked, leading to a reduction in middle ear fluid. However, many studies show that tonsillectomy does not affect the long-term course of otitis media.

The tonsils are essential lymphoid structures that play an important role in protecting the ear, nose, and throat area from bacteria and viruses that may gain entrance through the nose or mouth. Thus, removal of tonsils may increase susceptibility to infections of the ear, nose, and throat. There is even evidence that the incidence of bulbar paralysis from polio is greater (up to four times) in persons who have had their tonsils removed. In one report, 35 out of 39 cases of bulbar poliomyelitis had been tonsillectomized.[31, 32]

Adenoidectomy

The adenoids are lymphoid structures located near the tonsils and the opening of the eustachian tube. Removal of adenoids is performed to "unblock" the eustachian tube opening. A number of studies show that this procedure has no effect on middle ear fluid or infection, and has little effect on the long-term course of otitis media. This is especially true in children with a history of allergy.[33, 34, 35, 36]

The combined rates of tonsillectomy and adenoidectomy

was once as high as 1.2 million procedures per year. As the popularity of tympanostomy has grown, the use of tonsillectomy/adenoidectomy has fallen to below 580,000 per year.[37]

Myringotomy

Myringotomy is performed by making an incision in the eardrum. The purpose is to relieve pressure within the middle ear cavity and allow fluid to escape. Sometimes myringotomy is performed alone. It is also the first step taken before the insertion of tubes. As with other surgical procedures in otitis media, it has not been conclusively shown to be effective. Members of a medical consensus conference recently concluded that "no convincing data from clinical trials have been reported to support the value of myringotomy with or without antimicrobial therapy for acute otitis media." (They agreed that it may be of value for suppurative complications of otitis media and some other indications).[38] The only advantage of myringotomy appears to be pain relief, and this occurs in only a small percentage of children.[39]

One problem associated with myringotomy is that the incision in the eardrum often heals quickly. If the underlying disease has not been effectively treated, middle ear effusion quickly returns.[40]

In roughly one-fifth of all ear infections, the eardrum ruptures without intervention. Myringotomy is often used to prevent spontaneous rupture of the eardrum in the belief that an incision in the eardrum heals more efficiently than a rupture. However, ruptures usually heal completely within two weeks. Some doctors feel ruptures are not generally a cause for concern.[41]

Complications of Otitis Media

Temporary and permanent injury to structures within the middle ear chamber are among the possible complications of otitis media. These include: scarring of the eardrum; thickening of the eardrum; permanent rupture of the eardrum; growth of polyps, granules, or cholesteatoma (the formation of a cyst-like mass filled with cholesterol and cells); tympanosclerosis (see chapter 3); and hearing loss. These complications can occur with or without treatment, although adequate treatment usually reduces the likelihood of complications. There is evidence (discussed in chapter 3) that certain treatments may even encourage the development of some of the above complications.

One of the most common complications of otitis media is mastoiditis. The mastoid is part of the temporal bone and is located just behind the ear. Within the temporal bone reside all of the structures of the middle ear. When infection or inflammation of the middle ear becomes severe, it can spread into what are called the mastoid air cells. The signs of mastoiditis include:[42]

- Thick pus discharging from the middle ear.
- Ear pushed out with sagging of the ear canal.
- Redness over the mastoid process.
- Mastoid tenderness.
- Fever, headache.
- X-ray evidence of breakdown of the mastoid's cellular partitions.

These symptoms are not always present. According to Dr. C.R. Pfaltz, antibiotics have changed the course of mastoiditis. Many of the specific signs that used to be associated with mastoiditis are often masked by the use of antibiotics.[43]

Mastoiditis can be followed by other complications. The most common among these is meningitis, which results when an infection has spread from the mastoid to the covering of the brain known as the meninges. Meningitis is a serious illness that requires the immediate attention of a physician and antibiotic treatment. Symptoms of meningitis include:

- Headache.
- Neck stiffness.
- Lethargy.
- Sleepiness.

- Loss of appetite.
- Vomiting.
- Fever.
- Chills.

Incidentally, the incidence of meningitis due to *Haemophilus influenzae* (a common ear-infecting bacteria) has risen by several hundred percent in some parts of the country, in spite of the widespread use of antibiotics to treat otitis media.[44]

Other complications of otitis media include: brain abcess, sigmoid sinus thrombosis, and labyrinthitis. In a review of the complications of otitis media, Dr. Jack Froom states, ". . . fortunately [these complications] are very infrequent." When these complications occur, they usually require antibiotic or surgical intervention.[45]

*   *   *

Childhood otitis media is a complex problem. For many children, bouts of otitis occur and then resolve on their own within a short time. In other children, the process is more deeply rooted and requires intervention. As with any illness, there exists a potential for complications to develop. Prevention of complications is often the rationale given for the widespread use of antibiotics and surgery. However, antibiotics and surgery are not without complications of their own. In chapters 2 and 3, we will explore the side of the treatment story that is rarely told. That is, are antibiotics and tubes safe, and are they effective?

Chapter 2

Antibiotics:
Sensible Use or Abuse?

"It is no accident that the most allergic generation in history has been raised on antibiotics. Several times a week I see a new patient whose allergies appeared or became much worse after a course of antibiotics." [1]

Leo Galland, M.D.

The editor of the journal *Clinical Otolaryngology* once wrote that ". . . otitis media is a self-limiting disease, which is not affected by any of the current methods of treatment."[2] There are two important considerations in his statement. First, self-limiting means that a condition will usually run its course and improve over time. If otitis media is indeed self-limiting, are doctors justified in using the aggressive forms of antibiotic treatment we're accustomed to seeing? Second, if otitis media is not affected by current methods of treatment, does it not cast further doubt on the need for such extensive antibiotic use on children with otitis media?

To put this in perspective, consider the history of antibiotic use. At the time antibiotics were discovered, there were a number of serious infectious diseases that claimed the lives of hundreds of thousands of people. Infections from contagion and trauma were rendered seemingly impotent by the long-awaited miracle drugs called antibiotics. With their new-found arsenal, doctors slowly began to expand the use of antibiotics to include the treatment of bacterial diseases that were not life-threatening. Eventually antibiotics crept into use for almost any condition in which bacteria were thought to be involved. This included relatively minor conditions such as otitis media. We then saw the evolution (one might arguably call it regression) to prophylactic, or preventive antibiotic prescribing. In cases that were often of viral origin, children were given antibiotics to "prevent a secondary bacterial infection."

Prior to the antibiotic era, roughly 80 percent of all ear infections resolved spontaneously.[3] Today, nearly 9 out of 10 children diagnosed with middle ear infection will receive an antibiotic for their condition. Perhaps this antibiotic use is justified. Perhaps it's not.

In the management of any illness, doctors must always consider the so-called risk/benefit ratio. If a child suffers from middle ear infection, does he face a greater risk from the disease or the antibiotic? For decades, doctors were unquestioning in their belief that the risks of otitis media far outweighed the risk of antibiotics. Antibiotics were thought to be benevolent substances that imparted only good to the patient. However, we now know that antibiotics are a double-edged sword.

In spite of this knowledge, antibiotics are prescribed to children with more zeal today than ever before. From 1977 to 1986, antibiotic prescriptions to children under age 10 increased an alarming 51 percent, while the number of children in this age group grew by only 9 percent. In contrast, antibiotic prescriptions to the general population declined substantially during this time.[4]

According to Wendy Nelson, of the FDA's epidemiology and surveillance office, in 1977, 26 percent of all antibiotics were prescribed for otitis media. By 1986, the diagnosis of otitis media accounted for 42 percent of all antibiotics prescribed to pediatric outpatients. Antibiotic prescriptions to children under three showed the most dramatic increase.[5]

Amoxicillin, the most frequently prescribed drug for otitis media, now has the distinction of being the most frequently prescribed antibiotic of all—accounting for 21 percent of antibiotics used in 1986. A report published in *Medical World News* (1987) showed that, in the pediatric population, broad-spectrum penicillins and sulfa-containing drugs accounted for roughly 65 percent of all antibiotics prescribed in 1986.[6]

These figures provide reason for concern because of the potential hazards associated with the liberal use of antibacterial drugs. Among the most commonly cited problems with antibiotic use are:

- Antibiotic use can lead to the development of antibiotic-resistant bacteria.
- Antibiotics are associated with many adverse physical effects.
- There is conflicting information regarding whether antibiotics are effective for the majority of children with otitis media.
- There is uncertainty over the value of prophylactic (preventive) antibiotics.
- We don't fully understand the impact of the additional antibiotics children are exposed to through the food supply.

Parents need to take these issues seriously because not all doctors do.

Antibiotic-Resistant Bacteria

Indiscriminate use of antibiotics is leading us to one of the most frightening eras in recent memory. That is, the return of infectious diseases for which there is no cure. Two decades following the introduction of antibiotics, doctors began to observe an alarming trend. Infectious diseases that were once treatable no longer responded to antibiotics. Those that did respond often required five to ten times the amount of the drug that used to be effective. The reason—bacteria were developing resistance to the drugs.

In response to this surge in antibiotic-resistant bacteria, pharmaceutical researchers developed a new array of antibiotics against which the bacteria had no resistance. Over time, bacteria developed resistance to the new drugs as well. According to Dr. Marc Lappé in *When Antibiotics Fail*, by 1960 roughly 80 percent of the tested *staphylococcal* organisms showed resistance to penicillin, tetracycline, and chloramphenicol. Today, penicillin can kill only 10 percent of the varieties of *Staphylococcus aureus* that it used to dispose of easily.[7]

Gonorrhea was once easily cured with moderate doses of penicillin. Today, however, it takes several substantial doses of penicillin to cure the disease. More frightening is the number of resistant strains of gonorrhea that have popped up around the world that do not respond to penicillin at all.

The earliest association with antibiotic resistance and otitis media appeared in a paper entitled "The Increasing Incidence of Ampicillin-Resistant Haemophilus Influenzae: A Cause of Otitis Media." *Haemophilus influenzae* is one of the most commonly found bacteria in infected middle ear fluid. In this report, Dr. R. Schwartz and his colleagues observed that in 1975, only one ampicillin-resistant strain of *H. influenzae* was isolated from the middle ear fluid of children in their study. By 1976, 18 percent of all *H. influenzae* had become resistant to ampicillin. Midway through 1977, the percentage of ampicillin-resistant *H. influenzae* had grown to 35 percent— an almost 35 percent increase in just two years.[8]

This trend in bacterial development of antibiotic resistance is not unlike the increasing resistance of agricultural pests to pesticides. In 1938, scientists knew of just seven insect and mite species that had acquired resistance to pesticides. By 1984, that figure had climbed to 447 and included most of the world's major pests. In response to heavier pesticide use and a wider variety of pesticides, pests have evolved sophisticated mechanisms for resisting the action of chemicals designed to kill them.[9] Pesticides also kill the pests' natural enemies, much like antibiotics kill the natural enemies of harmful bacteria in the body.

Antibiotic resistance often develops in bacteria when they are repeatedly exposed to an antibiotic. Children who have received repeated courses of ampicillin, or other antibiotics in the penicillin group, harbor more antibiotic-resistant *Haemophilus influenzae* than those with little or no exposure to these drugs. Also, ampicillin-resistant strains of *H. influenzae* are reported more often in children with otitis media that is relapsing, recurrent, or chronic than in children with an initial infection.[10]

Not only do antibiotic-resistant bacteria pass the tools for resistance among their species, but from one species to another. This allows ampicillin-resistant *H. influenzae,* for example, to pass the gene for resistance (called an R-plasmid) to other *H. influenzae*, to common strep bacteria in the throat, to normal intestinal bacteria, or to any number of other organisms as well.

Antibiotic-resistant bacteria in the environment or the intestine also can pass on their tools for resistance. Consider the common intestinal bacteria *E. coli*. According the Dr. H.G. Welch, a specialist in the study of antibiotic resistance, *E. coli* is one of the most frequently resistant bacteria to both ampicillin and amoxicillin. This bacteria has the ability to pass the genes for resistance to either *H. influenzae* or *Streptococcus pneumoniae* —two common ear-infecting bacteria.

In *Postgraduate Medicine* (1984), Dr. Welch comments that ". . . antibiotic use, while contributing to the immediate demise of bacteria, serves to 'educate' microbes by establishing selective pressure that favors the 'smarter' bacteria, i.e., those that can resist the antibiotic."[11] Antibiotics such as ampicillin destroy susceptible *H. influenzae* in the middle ear, but the handful that remain are resistant to the drug. They reproduce and before long there is a large colony of resistant bacteria.

The consequences of antibiotic resistance can be serious. In one Minnesota hospital, patients who harbored antibiotic-resistant staph bacteria required hospitals stays 43 days longer than those with non-resistant staph. Those with resistant staph infections also had a higher mortality rate.[12] As this study shows, antibiotic resistance can lead to diseases that are not responsive to any form of therapy.

Haemophilus influenzae is a sobering example. This bacteria is not only associated with middle ear infection, but with meningitis and epiglottitis as well. Meningitis is a serious inflammation of the brain that must be treated with antibiotics. Epiglottitis is a serious and life-threatening disease that occurs when *H. influenzae* type b causes the epiglottis to swell, which closes off the airway, resulting in suffocation. (The epiglottis is a cartilaginous flap that prevents food and water from entering the lungs during swallowing.) It too must be treated vigorously and rapidly with antibiotics. However, if the bacteria are resistant to the antibiotic being used, the disease will not respond to treatment. Herein lies the most serious dilemma of antibiotic overuse. When life-threatening illness occurs, will the bacteria succumb to our drugs?

Adverse Physical Effects of Antibiotics

When antibiotics are used, there is often a trade-off between benefits and adverse physical effects. Sometimes the need for the antibiotic outweighs the risk of these physical effects, and the use of the drug is justified. When antibiotics are used excessively, the physical harm often offsets the benefits of the drug. Listed below are some adverse effects associated with antibiotics.

Destruction of Helpful Intestinal Bacteria
The common intestinal bacteria *Lactobacillus acidophilus* and *Bifidobacterium bifidus* are essential to proper digestive function, immune function, and synthesis of certain vitamins.[13] In

addition, they protect us from infections of the intestinal tract. Most antibiotics are undiscriminating with regard to intestinal bacteria. When antibiotics are used, *L. acidophilus* and *B. bifidus* are among the first to be killed. (The important functions of these bacteria are discussed in chapter 6.)

Increased Susceptibility to Intestinal Infection

Because of the adverse effect on *L. acidophilus*, *B. bifidus*, and the local immune system, antibiotics can cause children to be more susceptible to parasitic infection. For instance, infection by the parasite *Giardia lamblia* is made easier following the administration of antibiotics. *G. lamblia* is one of the most common waterborne parasites in the United States, affecting an estimated 18 million people.[14] *Giardia* is also listed among the top ten most common infectious agents found in day care centers.[15] In addition to the intestinal problems created, parasitic infection causes immune suppression, which often leads to increased susceptibility to subsequent bacterial infection.[16]

Antibiotic use also can result in an overgrowth of the bacterium *Clostridium dificile* in the colon. This has been linked with the development of a painful inflammatory condition known as pseudomembranous colitis.[17]

A yeast organism that normally lives in the intestinal tract—and is kept in check by *L. acidophilus* and *B. bifidus*—overgrows following excessive antibiotic use. This yeast, called *Candida albicans*, is responsible for the development of food allergy, environmental sensitivity, and recurring infections.[18] *Candida albicans* also adds to intestinal problems by stimulating the growth of *Giardia lamblia*.[19]

The ability of antibiotics to increase susceptibility to intestinal parasites is a serious matter because parasitic infection of children in the United States is a growing problem. In one study of 321 children from Houston, Texas, 49.5 percent tested positive for intestinal parasites. The rate of infection is high in Houston in part because of its proximity to Mexico. However, the rate of parasitic infection of children in the general population is increasing nationwide. It is especially high in the Southwestern United States.[20]

Irritation of the Intestinal Lining

Some antibiotics can cause a thinning of the lining of the intestinal tract. This often leads to inflammation and poor absorption of vitamins, minerals, and fats. Disruption of the intestinal lining causes the permeability of the intestine to change, resulting in the development of food allergy.

Inhibition of Immunity

Antibiotics can inhibit the ability of white blood cells (called neutrophils) to protect against the overgrowth of *Candida albicans*.[21] Once an infestation of *Candida albicans* gets out of control, multiple health problems typically follow. Children who have had repeated doses of antibiotics for recurrent otitis media, but have failed to improve, often suffer from a secondary problem caused by *Candida albicans*. Under these circumstances, further antibiotic use severely aggravates the situation. Usually such children will not improve until antibiotics are discontinued and the yeast problems are addressed.

Some antibiotics prevent neutrophil chemotaxis.[22] Whenever an infectious agent is present in the body, chemical signals are sent out that tell the white blood cells where to go, a process called chemotaxis.

When white blood cells do get to the site of infection, they often release peroxides (such as hydrogen peroxide) that essentially "bleach" the bacteria to death. Some antibiotics reduce the ability of white blood cells to destroy bacteria in this way.[23]

Antibiotics can also depress natural killer cell activity and reduce the production of antibodies.[24] The depressed antibody production is important since antibodies are produced in response to a bacteria as a means of signaling the body to kill it. Antibodies also provide a "memory" of invading bacteria. With this memory in place, the likelihood of succumbing to future infection by that bacteria is sharply reduced. When the memory is not sufficient, reinfection is more likely. Some antibiotics delay the antibody response. Frequently, the delay may last for up to 20 days after the antibiotic has been discontinued.[25]

Penicillin has been associated with a 1,000-fold increase of intestinal bacteria such as *E. coli* in the cecum (a pouch where the small and large intestine meet). Oral administration of penicillin for only four days can disrupt the normal ecology of the gut and cause *E. coli* and other bacteria to migrate to the lymph nodes within the mesentery (part of the abdominal lymph system). The mesenteric lymph nodes are an essential part of the immune system of the abdominal cavity.[26]

Reduced Absorption of Nutrients

There is some evidence that certain antibiotics reduce the absorption of nutrients such as vitamin K, vitamin B12, folic acid, calcium, and magnesium.[27] These effects may be minimal in children who are healthy or when antibiotic therapy is short-term. However, children who receive repeated doses of antibiotics or who suffer intestinal symptoms (such as diarrhea) from antibiotic therapy may experience losses of nutrients that can impair their ability to fight infection. The adverse affects of antibiotics on nutrients is likely to be greatest when: 1) broad-spectrum antibiotics are used, 2) repeated courses of antibiotics are used, 3) prophylactic or preventive antibiotics are used, and 4) the child has a history of malabsorption or intestinal disease.

Recently, a respected colleague of mine described the adverse antibiotic reaction experienced by one of her children. At age two, her son had been given a 10-day course of antibiotic for a middle ear infection. Shortly after beginning the drug, the boy experienced diarrhea and behavior changes. The diarrhea worsened and persisted for a total of seven weeks, at which time he began to develop paralysis of the right leg, arm, and eye. The paralysis remained, prompting my colleague to take her child to a neurologist. She told the doctor that her son's paralysis had come about following antibiotic therapy. The neurologist commented that this is somewhat common and that he saw about two of these cases per month.

Since I have found no evidence of this in the medical literature, it is difficult to say to what extent this type of reaction occurs. Yet to this boy the reaction was very real. Now at age ten, although improved, he continues to suffer impairment.

Antibiotics and Otitis Media: Helpful for Most Children?

There is evidence suggesting that antibiotics are effective in managing some types of middle ear infections. Members of a 1984 conference entitled "Controversies in Antimicrobial Agents for Otitis Media," chaired by Charles D. Bluestone, M.D., suggest that antimicrobial therapy *is* indicated for acute otitis media. Sulfonamides have been shown to be somewhat effective in treating ear infections.[28] Amoxicillin was found, in one trial, to be more effective than placebo in treating acute otitis media.[29] Researchers in Canada, after a study of 142 children, concluded that penicillin and ampicillin were superior to symptomatic therapy.[30] However, the percentage of children for whom antibiotics are useful may be low when compared with the number of children receiving antibiotics for otitis media. Supporting the latter contention are several studies conducted over the past two decades.

In a study of 2,975 children, two Dutch physicians, using a method called the "antibiotic timing treatment," set out to determine the effect of early *vs.* late *vs.* no antibiotic therapy in acute otitis media. Antibiotics were used only when signs of complications were threatening or present. In their study, 1,680 patients were treated with antibiotics and 1,367 were treated without antibiotics. The following conclusions were reached.[31]

1. 88 percent of all patients with acute otitis media *never* need antibiotics. [emphasis mine]

2. When antibiotics are begun on the first day of the disease, the frequency of recurrence is 2.9 times higher than when no antibiotics are used. When antibiotics are begun after the eighth day, the rate of recurrence is 1.3 times higher.

3. Antibiotic therapy does not shorten the disease by any standard.

4. Antibiotics should be reserved for cases in which complications are threatening or present.

5. When this approach is used, the rate of complications (e.g., mastoiditis) is low (0.3/1,000).

Numerous other studies performed in the United States and Scandinavia appear to support these findings. In cases of acute otitis media, conventional treatment consists of a 10-day course of antibiotics. However, roughly 50 percent of children receiving antibiotics continue to have otitis media with effusion after 10 to 14 days.[32, 33, 34] Doctors reporting on a recent study of 3,660 children in nine countries found that treatment with antibiotics had little impact on the rate of recovery.* In fact, those not given antibiotics experienced a slightly higher rate of recovery than those who received antibiotics.[35]

Many doctors have attributed the relatively high rate of antibiotic failure to the fact that parents do not give the antibiotic frequently enough or for the prescribed length of time. But is this a fact or an assumption? Prior to 1981, only one study had sought to prove whether full antibiotic compliance had any bearing on the course of otitis media. In 1981, Dr. Richard

---

*The authors urge caution in the interpretation of this study since some variables were not controlled. Still, they expressed great concern over the implications of their findings. (*British Medical Journal,* March, 1990)

Schwartz attempted to clarify this issue in a study of 105 children. His group concluded that "good pharmacologic [antibiotic] compliance will not reduce the frequency of otitis media with effusion found after treatment for acute otitis media," and that "the frequency of otitis media with effusion in compliant children *did not differ* from that found in non-compliant children."[36]

Doctors in the United States almost always prescribe antibiotics for 10 days when treating ear infections. No one is sure where this practice originated since there is no evidence in the medical literature that shows taking an antibiotic for this length of time is optimum. In fact, recent studies have shown that the results obtained following seven-day, five-day, three-day, or even two-day courses of antibiotics are comparable to those obtained when a 10-day course is prescribed. These shortened antibiotic regimens appear to carry no greater risk of complications from otitis media than the customary 10-day regimen.[37, 38, 39, 40]

Two important questions in assessing the value of antibiotics are: do they improve the symptoms of middle ear infection, and do they prevent recurrence of the infection? In 1981, Dr. F.L. Van Buchem and his associates studied 171 children and compared antibiotics only, myringotomy only, both antibiotics and myringotomy, and no treatment.

Van Buchem's group found that at one, two, and six months, children receiving the treatments fared no better in terms of pain, level of hearing, recurrence, fever, and healing time—the most important indicators for assessing progress of the disease—than did those not receiving treatment.[41] Though Van Buchem's study did not include seriously ill children, his findings are noteworthy.

Do antibiotics prevent recurrent ear infections? Dr. Michael Persico showed that when antibiotic therapy is begun early and frequently, the result is "*more* recurrent acute otitis media, less immune response, more side effects, allergy, and super infection."[42] Persico contends that the temporary sterilization of the middle ear often leads to an immediate reappearance of pathogenic bacteria, especially when the eustachian tube is not functioning (which is believed to be the case in many children).[43] These sentiments are echoed by M. M. Paparella, M.D., who states that "otitis media with effusion . . . appears to be more common *since* the widespread use of antibiotics."[44]

A 1987 report in *Pediatric Infectious Disease Journal* seems to support this view. When antibiotics are prescribed early, or immediately, for infection, the incidence of recurrent episodes is higher than when antibiotics are given later or not at all.[45] It appears that when treatment is delayed, children are able to develop natural immunity, thereby insulating them from future episodes. Early antibiotic therapy appears to inhibit the initial immune response.

Doctors have long equated killing bacteria with treating disease. But few physicians acknowledge that, while effective at eradicating microbes in the short term, antibiotics do nothing to correct underlying problems or contribute to tissue repair. Dr. L.E. Cluff, in *Clinical Concepts of Infectious Disease*, states, "Once injury from infection occurs, elimination of the microbes may prevent further injury; but return to normality is dependent upon other events. *Antibiotics cannot resolve inflammation, tissue necrosis, or pathophysiological processes*" [emphasis mine].[46] Doctors who simply treat an ear infection with antibiotics, and do nothing else, are likely overlooking important physiological happenings within the child's body that are signaling weakness. Unless these weaknesses are addressed (whether they be nutritional, environmental, or otherwise), full recovery cannot be expected to take place in the middle ear.

Preventing Complications

Among the most common arguments in favor of antibiotics is that they have reduced the rate of complications (such as mastoiditis and meningitis) encountered in otitis media. This is a reasonable assertion with which most doctors would agree.

However, Dutch researcher F.L. Van Buchem, M.D., contends that "no conclusion can be drawn, from the published work, on the influence of antibiotics on the incidence of mastoiditis."[47] In spite of the great advances in antibiotic therapy, there has been an increase ranging from 3 to 400 percent (based on studies in the United States, Canada, England, and Denmark) in the incidence of *Haemophilus influenzae* meningitis.[48]

Dr. C.R. Pfaltz reports that "antibiotics have changed the course of otitis media" because they can mask the development of more serious underlying disease. He says that antibiotics are of great importance when mastoiditis occurs, due to their ability to eliminate the bacterial infection within the middle ear. But antibiotics do not affect the inflammation within the mastoid process.[49] Still, most doctors believe antibiotics are a necessary tool in preventing complications.

Proper Use?

A final question surrounding the effectiveness of antibiotics is their proper use. In other words, is the correct drug given in the correct dosage? Are antibiotics indicated at all? One hospital study of antibiotic usage found that in 64 percent of the cases where antibiotics were used, their use was either not indicated or they were improperly administered in terms of drugs or dosage.[50] In 1975, the American Academy of Pediatrics recommended that tetracycline not be given to children under eight years of age (because it was found to cause liver damage, retarded bone growth, digestive disturbance, and permanently stained teeth). Yet a study in 1977 showed that 27 percent of physicians surveyed continued to give tetracycline to children under age eight, despite warnings.[51]

An unfortunate phenomenon occurs when doctors prescribe drugs more in an effort to satisfy the parents of an ailing child than out of clinical indication. An article in the *Wall Street Journal* describes a recent experiment by investigators from Harvard Medical School. ". . . 141 randomly chosen doctors, who were moderate to heavy prescribers of three particular drugs, received mailed information indicating that these drugs were ineffective or far more expensive than equally effective alternatives. They also received two follow-up visits in which specially-trained pharmacists discussed the clinical evidence with them."

"Almost half the doctors said they were merely satisfying their patients' demands for these drugs and indicated fears that *failure to meet such demands would risk losing patients* to more obliging physicians. Many conceded that the *prescribing couldn't be justified on scientific grounds*. Another quarter of the doctors cited a 'placebo' effect as justification. Writing a prescription, they argued, can have positive psychological benefit for the patients and thus possibly bring some relief" [emphasis mine].[52]

Accuracy of diagnosis is one final area of concern regarding the proper use of antibiotics. In order to recommend proper treatment, doctors must first make an accurate diagnosis of a child's condition. But doctors are not always certain of their diagnosis. Researchers from the International Primary Care Network found that doctors were certain of their diagnosis of otitis media in only 58 percent of children under twelve months.[53] This finding is of great concern since many children in which the diagnosis was uncertain undoubtedly received antibiotics. The low degree of diagnostic certainty is not necessarily the fault of doctors since children under twelve months are often difficult to examine. Yet, it adds to the dilemma of deciding when antibiotics are appropriate for children with otitis media.*

Preventive (Prophylactic) Antibiotics

Many doctors prescribe prophylactic antibiotics in the hope that an impending infection might be prevented. At first glance the practice seems rational. Marc Lappé, Ph.D., professor at

---

*Diagnostic certainty in children aged 13 to 30 months was 66 percent and 73 percent in those older than 30 months.

the University of Illinois, contends that prophylactic use of antibiotics comprises the "worst category of misuse."[54] He cites numerous studies that show 50 to 65 percent of prophylactically prescribed antibiotics are given innapropriately. According to Silverman and Lee in *Pills, Profit and Politics* (1974), ". . . the best thing that can be said about prophylactic antibiotics is that in most instances it is not clinically justifiable. It presents needless risks and unnecessary expense. At worst, it may be fatal for the patient."

Dr. Michael Persico and his associates found that prophylactic use of penicillin improved the clinical condition of recurrent acute otitis media. However, in the children who experienced a reduction in recurrent acute otitis media, there was no decrease in middle ear fluid. At all stages of follow-up, *there was no difference in middle ear appearance in those children* receiving prophylactic doses of penicillin when compared with those receiving a short course of ampicillin.[55] According to Dr. M. Tos, "Antibiotic treatment does not promote the development of secretory otitis, but is probably unable to prevent it."[56]

A recent report showed that prophylactic doses of antibiotics* prescribed at night for several months reduced the frequency of recurrent episodes of otitis media. The beneficial effects appeared to be most significant for children under age two and children attending day care. This is encouraging. However, the degree to which middle ear effusion had declined after six months was nearly the same in the placebo group as in the antibiotic groups.[57]

There may be instances where prophylactic antibiotics are required. However, because of the numerous adverse effects associated with indiscriminate antibiotic use, children chosen for prophylactic antibiotics should be selected carefully. In the

---

*Amoxicillin and sulfamethoxazole with trimethoprim were compared with placebo in this study. (*American Journal of Diseases of Children*, 1989)

world of antibiotics and bacteria, a cavalier attitude toward prescribing is no longer acceptable.

Foodborne Antibiotics

The clinical use of antibiotics is unfortunately not our only source of exposure. Agricultural antibiotic sales account for nearly three-fourths of all antibiotics sold in the United States (243 million dollars annually by 1979).[58] The use of antibiotics has been reported on more than 90 percent of the beef, pork, and poultry in the U.S. Drug-resistant *Salmonella* are appearing in tainted beef, poultry, and milk at an increasing rate. The total incidence of disease transmission due to tainted food is unknown, since many mild intestinal symptoms go unreported, and tracing an outbreak to its source is costly and difficult.

According to Dr. Richard Novick, farm animals contribute between 99 and 99.9 percent of all the resistant coliform bacteria (especially *E. coli*) in the environment. In addition, he states that there are no barriers to the spread of genes for antibiotic resistance and that they pose "a substantial hazard to human health due to therapeutic compromise."[59]

In 1983, a midwestern outbreak of intestinal disease in 18 people was associated with an antibiotic-resistant form of *Salmonella newport* (resistant to ampicillin, carbenicillin, and tetracycline). The source of the infection was traced to hamburger in which chlortetracycline had been used for growth promotion. (The use of this antibiotic led to the development of antibiotic-resistant *S. newport*.) Twelve of the people had been taking penicillin-derived antibiotics in the 24- to 48-hour period before the onset of intestinal symptoms.

According to scientists at the State Health Departments in Minnesota and North Dakota, the patients had been infected before they took antibiotics. Their use of antibiotics, to which the *S. newport* was resistant, led to a reduction in the normal intestinal bacteria, resulting in more serious intestinal infection by *S. newport*.

Researchers in charge of this case conclude that ". . . anti-microbial-resistant organisms of animal origin cause serious human illness," and urge ". . . *far more prudent use of anti-microbials in both human beings* and animals" [emphasis mine].[60]

Antibiotics are used in animal feed to slightly enhance growth (by 5 to 6 percent). However, animals raised on anti-biotic-treated feed serve as a reservoir of antibiotic-resistant bacteria. Over the years, scientists have observed a direct rela-tionship between the number of resistant strains of bacteria appearing in animals and the use of antibiotics in animal feed. These antibiotic-resistant bacteria have appeared on meat and dairy products sold to consumers. When these products are consumed, the bacteria are passed into the intestinal tract of those who eat them. This is believed to be partially responsible for the increase in antibiotic-resistant bacteria in humans.

Antibiotic-resistant bacteria in our food is unfortunately not the only hazard associated with agricultural use of antibio-tics. The drugs themselves are making their way into the food we feed our children. In 1988, the antibiotic sulfamethazine appeared in 25 percent of all milk consumed by Americans. Sulfamethazine has shown up in illegal levels in 5 to 15 per-cent of the pork sold to consumers in recent years and 1 to 3 percent of the veal.

The FDA allows up to 100 ppb sulfamethazine in meat prior to slaughter. This drug is illegal for use in lactating dairy cows. No prescription is required to purchase sulfamethazine. The FDA merely requires that farmers not give it to hogs, poul-try, and cattle for several days before slaughter. Unfortunately, enforcement is minimal, and illegal residues are commonplace.[61]

In December of 1989, the FDA issued a statement of its intent to ban the use of sulfamethazine in animals by the year 1990. However, the pharmaceutical industry is poised to oppose this ban, and as it has shown in the past, it is capable of winning.

The European Economic Community has recently banned the use of tetracycline and other antibiotics in all animals.

Moreover, they have threatened to ban the import of U.S. meat and dairy products in which antibiotics (or hormones) have been used. Hopefully this will bring about change in the U.S. practices.

Agricultural use of antibiotics results in drug residue and antibiotic-resistant bacteria in the food we eat. The effect of this type of low-grade, long-term exposure on children (or adults) is unclear. What is clear is that our use of antibiotics in medicine must take this additional exposure into account. You as a consumer of food should demand, through your purchasing power, that only antibiotic-free meat and milk be available. This can be done by purchasing food that is labeled organic or raised free of antibiotics. As consumers of health care, you should demand that your doctors give good rationale for their use of antibiotics on your child.

In Support of Antibiotics

This chapter is not written as a full-fledged assault on the use of antibiotics. The intent is to show parents and health care professionals the hazards of unbridled use of these drugs. No one desires to go back to the pre-antibiotic era when infectious diseases were rampant. But in our zeal to eradicate microbes at all costs, we may have unwittingly chosen the very course we have sought to avoid.

Antibiotics, when used wisely, are an extremely valuable weapon in the medical arsenal. When microorganisms threaten to overwhelm the defenses of a sick child, antibiotics should be used. When complications are present or imminent, antibiotics should be used. There are numerous circumstances under which prudent antibiotic use is to be considered in the management of otitis media and other diseases. Whether they are necessary for the treatment of your child can only be decided after careful consideration of the facts and consultation with your doctor.

If your doctor chooses to prescribe antibiotics, I believe

it is essential that he or she also address dietary, nutritional, and other factors discussed in this book. When these factors are addressed, the effectiveness of any treatment should be enhanced, and the risk of recurrent infection reduced.

Chapter 3

Tubes: Effectiveness, Hazards, and Complications

*"Incredibly, one of the side effects of this procedure, performed to cure recurrent otitis media, is **acute** otitis media."* [1]
Robert S. Mendelsohn, M.D.

Tympanostomy, or insertion of tubes in the eardrum, has rapidly emerged as the surgical method of choice in the treatment of childhood ear infections. Recent estimates show that tympanostomy is performed on more than one million children each year,[2] at an average cost of 800 to 1,000 dollars per surgery. In many cases the surgery is performed on both ears, resulting in perhaps almost two million tubes annually. It is common for tubes to fall out prematurely, often within 4 to 7 months.[3, 4] The recurrence of middle ear effusion following the rejection of tubes seems to occur in as high as 40 percent of all children. Of the children who prematurely reject their tubes, 33 to 75 percent require a second surgery to replace them.[5, 6]

There is disagreement over whether tubes are effective, and if so, when their use should be considered. Most otolaryngologists resort to tubes in one to two months when antibiotics are unsuccessful in resolving a case of otitis media. Yet, in one survey, 40 percent of otolaryngologists felt that tubes were used too frequently.[7, 8]

How It's Done

A child is first placed under general anesthesia. The surgeon locates the ideal spot on the eardrum for placement of the tube and makes an incision. A tiny tube is then placed through the opening. Tubes vary in size, material and design, but are basically similar. The term tympanostomy derives its meaning from the words tympanum, which is the middle ear cavity, and ostomy, which refers to any surgery in which an artificial opening is formed.

The Rationale

Doctors generally recommend tubes after antibiotics have failed to clear up a recurring earache. The hope is that tubes will:

- Reduce middle ear pressure.
- Allow fluid to drain from the middle ear.
- Restore hearing.
- Prevent permanent hearing damage.
- Prevent recurring ear infections.

Tubes are able to reduce middle ear pressure, allow fluid to drain, and improve hearing in the short term (1-3 months). But whether tubes can prevent long-term hearing loss or prevent recurrent otitis is a source of controversy. Moreover, there is a great likelihood that the underlying disease is unaffected. Most doctors agree that eustachian tube dysfunction is at the root of otitis media, yet there is evidence that tympanostomy does nothing to affect eustachian tube function.[9]

Effectiveness and Complications

According to Dr. Gunnar B. Stickler, of the Department of Pediatrics at the Mayo Clinic, the use of tubes has not been adequately tested to support its widespread use. He states in a commentary in the journal *Pediatrics* (1984) that the best prescription for otitis media is a "tincture of time." He goes on to say, ". . . many of us in practice today had fluid in our ears when we were children. Did it really cause a degree of retardation? If not, let us declare a moratorium on tube placements until solid data supporting the procedure have been reported."[10]

Several controlled studies of tympanostomy have been reported. In Volume 71 of the *Journal of the Royal Society of Medicine*,[11] Dr. M.J. Brown and his colleagues reported a study of 60 children with bilateral otitis media. Both ears were determined by culture to be infected. Tympanostomy tubes, or grommets (as they're known in Great Britain), were placed in one ear while leaving the other ear to chance. After five years of follow-up, his group concluded that:

1. Within the first six months, hearing gains are somewhat better with insertion of tubes.

2. After six months, there is no difference between the two ears.

3. At five years, there is no statistical difference in the incidence of fluid in the grommet ear as compared with the control.

4. There was a 13 percent incidence of scars in the grommet ear compared with zero in the control.

5. At five years, there was a 42 percent incidence of **tympanosclerosis**, in the grommet ear, compared with zero in the control. Tympanosclerosis is a condition where masses of hard, dense, connective tissue surround the bones (auditory ossicles) in the middle ear.[12]

Tympanosclerosis is a progressive phenomenon. The incidence increases over time to as much as 65 percent at 3-4 years after insertion of the tube.[13] Dr. T. Lildholt found tympanosclerosis to occur in 77 percent of children with tubes.[14]

These studies and others show that the use of tubes (or myringotomy) leads to some degree of tympanosclerosis. Some researchers suggest that tympanosclerosis is due to the effects of the ear infection itself rather than an injury resulting from tubes. They contend that if left untreated, the ears would develop tympanosclerosis anyway.[15] However, Dr. Brown and his colleagues point out that the control ears in their study received no tubes, and they developed no tympanosclerosis. For this reason Brown concludes that "the myringotomy and grommet insertion were the offending agents."[16]

Drs. Kilby, Richards, and Hart, in a two-year follow-up study comparing tympanostomy and myringotomy in 54 children, concluded that tubes do not alter the long-term course of otitis media. They report that eardrum scars, with membrane thickening, were three times more frequent in the ears receiving tubes than in the ears receiving simple myringotomy.[17]

In another study, tympanostomy and adenoidectomy were compared in 58 children suffering from mucoid middle ear effusion. Of those children receiving adenoidectomy, only 20.7 percent had normal hearing and clear middle ears during a two-year follow-up. Following tympanostomy, only 59 percent had normal hearing after two years. What is important here is the finding that in children with allergy, both tympanostomy and adenoidectomy yield "similarly poor results."[18] (See chapter 5.)

There do seem to be some short-term benefits to tympanostomy in some children with chronic secretory otitis media. In 1984, 54 children with bilateral chronic secretory otitis media (who failed to respond to antibiotic therapy) were treated by placement of a tube into just one ear. The two ears were then compared for degree of improvement. At three months, the side with the tube improved significantly. However, at one year, there was no significant difference between the two sides.[19] In a 1985 study of 116 children with chronic otitis media, Drs. N. Yanagihara and T. Yagi found that 46 percent accepted tubes without problems. These investigators concluded that insertion of tubes is a valuable method of treating ears under certain conditions.[20]

From the evidence available in 1985, Heinz Eichenwald, M.D., concluded that ". . . tympanostomy—now one of the most frequently performed surgical procedures in the United States—not only often fails to achieve its aim of reducing the frequency of episodes of acute otitis media, *but may be associated with a long-term risk of hearing loss*" [emphasis mine].[21]

Tympanostomy also carries a risk of infectious complications. Fred Herzon, M.D., reports that otorrhea (pus drainage from the middle ear outward through the tube) is a frequent and often underconsidered consequence of tympanostomy. In his study of 140 patients, 21 percent experienced post-surgical infections. Most children required follow-up therapy with antibiotics. Almost four percent of these infections were serious and complicated, necessitating multiple courses of antibiotics.[22] Dr. George A. Gates and his colleagues at the University of Texas Health Science-San Antonio have shown that the risk of one or more episodes of otorrhea after placement of tubes is three times greater than after simple myringotomy.[23]

When a tube is placed into the eardrum, an open passage to the outside is formed. The open tube is believed to allow bacteria,[24] viruses, and allergens to migrate into the middle ear cavity. This increases the chance for reinfection of the middle ear.

Complications of tympanostomy include: [25, 26]

- Anesthetic risks (one death per 5,000 to 10,000 procedures).
- Psychological trauma.
- Postsurgical infection.

- Localized foreign body reaction (reaction to the presence of the tube).

- Granulation (formation of small granules of tissue).

- Hyalinization (conversion of tissue into a glass-like substance).

- Tympanosclerosis (formation of hard, dense tissue around the bones of the middle ear).

- Hearing loss (temporary or permanent, varying degrees).

- Persistent perforation of the eardrum.

- Dislocation of tube into the middle ear cavity.

- Blockage of the tube rendering it ineffective.

The combined rates of the above complications, up to eight years from the time of tube insertion, range from 32 to 60 percent.[27, 28] The rate of complications associated with the placement of tubes goes up proportionately with the length of time the tubes remain in place.

It is important to realize that tubes are not designed to cure otitis media. They are intended as intermediate measures used to drain fluid from the middle ear and restore hearing (short-term). Since tubes do not affect the underlying disease process, they are likely to be ineffective as a sole therapy for many children.

Even the most ardent opponents of tympanostomy acknowledge that the procedure has value under the right circumstances. Based on the evidence, I think it can be safely argued that tympanostomy does not hold the potential for benefit that some doctors contend. There may be a substantial number of children who receive tubes unnecessarily. In chapter 5, we'll explore the causes of otitis media. After seeing the multiplicity of factors that contribute to otitis media, it will be obvious that more than tubes is required to correct the underlying problems that lead up to otitis media. Doctors who recommend tubes should make every effort to address these underlying weaknesses while the tubes are in place.

Chapter 4

Hearing Loss and Delayed Development: Myth or Reality?

Who shall decide when doctors disagree?

Alexander Pope

Parents are rightfully concerned about the prospects of otitis media leading to hearing loss in their children. The added possibility of intellectual impairment, resulting from prolonged hearing loss, has caused parents and doctors to perceive otitis media as a serious and dreaded condition that requires rigorous therapy. Yet over the years, conflicting research has made the issue of otitis media, hearing loss, and delayed development a confusing one.

Normal hearing occurs when sound waves travel from their source to the eardrum. The eardrum vibrates, setting the ear ossicles—bones of the middle ear—in motion. Vibration of the ear ossicles causes vibration of a fluid within the *inner* ear. This fluid passes over tiny hairlike structures that connect to nerve fibers. These fibers conduct impulses to the part of the nervous system where sound is perceived.

Proper function of the eardrum is dependent upon the pressure being equal on both sides. Equal pressure is accomplished by the eustachian tube opening and closing, according to the external pressure. Consider the pressure you feel in your ears when riding in an elevator or traveling up a mountain road. The rapid change in altitude results in a change in atmospheric pressure, causing a change in the pressure exerted on the eardrum from the outside. Swallowing or yawning generally opens the eustachian tube sufficiently to allow air to rush in or out of the middle ear, thus equalizing the internal and external pressure on the eardrum. It is these constant adjustments to the changing external environment that allow the eardrum to function normally under almost any condition. Normal function of the ear ossicles is dependent upon the same conditions. In order for them to conduct sound properly, they require an "air-filled" or aerated environment. This is also accomplished by the eustachian tube.

Any interference with the vibration of either the eardrum or middle ear ossicles can lead to a decrease in hearing acuity. This is precisely what occurs during middle ear infection or inflammation. When fluid or pus accumulates in the middle ear, pressure is exerted outward on the eardrum, causing it to be fixed and rigid. In the fluid-filled environment, the ear ossicles no longer vibrate freely. The combination of these two factors leads to decreased *conduction* of sound waves and impaired hearing ability. Another common contributor to decreased hearing is congestion within the nasal cavity, which obstructs the opening of the eustachian tube, preventing the middle ear from being properly aerated. This leads to increased pressure within the middle ear, a feeling of fullness, and sometimes pain. The above type of hearing deficiency is known as **conductive hearing loss** and is the most common form associated with otitis media.

Another form of hearing loss is less common and more serious. It is known as **sensorineural hearing loss** and occurs when there has been residual damage to nerves and structures of the inner ear. This form of hearing loss is more likely to occur in children with chronic recurrent otitis media or otitis media that is untreated.

There is no disagreement over whether otitis media leads to temporary losses in hearing. Hearing changes in children with acute otitis media are usually short-lived, lasting only weeks to months. Children with chronic recurrent otitis media often experience hearing difficulty that is longer-lasting. Yet in most cases, the hearing impairment suffered by these children is modest and generally not sufficient even to interfere with ordinary communication.[1, 2] Whether otitis media leads to permanent hearing impairment is another question.

Robert S. Mendelsohn, M.D., has long contended that ear infections do not lead to permanent hearing loss. In *The People's Doctor*, he states, "If a high percentage of untreated ear infections were to result in hearing loss, the incidence of deafness in children would be staggering, since many ear infections are undetected by the mother, undetected by a physician, inadequately treated (since not all patients take the prescribed amount of medication), and often not checked afterward to see whether they have disappeared. In some school screening tests, when children with a loss of hearing acuity were tested some months later, with no intervening treatment, they showed normal levels of hearing."[3]

The issues upon which some controversy rest are whether changes in hearing lead to developmental delays, and if so, whether the delays are permanent.

Several recent studies have suggested that there is *no* link between early childhood ear infections and developmental delays. Dr. Denzil Brooks, in a 1986 study of 80 children, concluded that "no correlations were found to support the hypothesis that middle ear dysfunction during the early years of schooling is causally related to poor academic achievement."[4] A study published in the journal *Pediatrics* in 1986 also found no correlation between poor academic performance and early childhood otitis media.[5]

For every study that shows no link between otitis media, hearing loss, and delayed development, there appears to be a study that confirms a link. In a review of the medical literature, Dr. C.R. Kirkwood states that "all studies reviewed show a strong correlation between otitis media and learning disabilities, with children with learning disabilities having several times the incidence of otitis media of controls."[6] However, in response to this argument, some researchers contend that the possibility exists that other underlying factors, common to both otitis media and learning disability, may be responsible for the correlation.*[7]

Many studies that show an association between otitis media and developmental impairments have relied on parental recall, which is not viewed widely as a reliable means of assessment. According to one researcher, several studies dealt with children referred to a clinic *because* of academic underachievement.[8, 9]

Even if there were evidence to support a direct link between otitis media and delayed intellectual development, the question remains whether the developmental delays are permanent. This was addressed in a study of elementary school children who had previously been tested and found to have hearing impairment and poor language performance. The results of a five-year follow-up of these children, published in the *British Journal of Audiology*, found that their hearing had improved substantially and their academic performance was on a par with their peers.[10]

While direct links to intellectual impairment have been difficult to prove, there is evidence of behavioral changes developing in children whose earaches are long-standing. In one study, 44 children were followed for three years after birth

---

*For example, scientists estimate that 20 to 30 percent of children under age six have unacceptably high levels of lead in their bodies. Lead is a known inhibitor of immune function and can increase a child's susceptibility to infection. Lead also contributes to hearing problems and learning disability. It is conceivable that a percentage of children who suffer from recurrent otitis media, hearing problems, and learning problems do so as result of lead toxicity. (To my knowledge, this relationship has not been thoroughly studied.) A principal cause of lead toxicity in children is inhalation and ingestion of lead-laden dust from leaded house paint. This is a very serious problem. See chapter 7 for more information on lead.

and assessed for cognitive and academic performance. No correlation was found between early childhood otitis media with effusion and these measures of academic achievement. However, it was learned that the children with more otitis media with effusion ". . . tended to be described by their teachers as less task-oriented and less able to work independently."[11] The children in this study were all in day care, which puts them at greater risk to developing otitis media. They were also socioeconomically disadvantaged, which puts them at greater risk both to otitis media and to delayed intellectual development.

Evidently, controversy still surrounds the issue of hearing loss and delayed development. The absence of a direct link is important because some doctors base their rationale for treatment (especially surgical) on the "threat" of potential permanent hearing loss and delayed development. On this, J.L. Paradise, M.D. comments "What seems *not* reasonable, however, is to subject largely asymptomatic infants or young children with middle-ear effusions to surgical intervention relatively early in the course of their illness, i.e., less than two to three months after onset, invoking as sole justification the fear of later developmental handicaps."[12]

This does not imply that children with otitis media should go untreated or that those with hearing loss should be ignored. Despite the existence of conflicting evidence, audiologists have expressed alarm over the growing number of preschool children who are minimally hearing impaired. Many feel that recurrent otitis media impacts adversely upon learning, speech, behavior, and even interaction with peers.

According to Lilian Rojas, Ph.D., a speech, hearing, and language specialist, aphasiologist, and international consultant to educational institutions, all persons who work with children, from physicians to educators, must be made aware of the potential problems facing children with hearing deficits. Dr. Rojas cites evidence that there are critical stages of development that can be delayed by the presence of persistent middle ear effusion. She states that in some children with middle ear effusion, hearing may fall within the normal decibel range but the quality of sound perception may suffer. Hearing may seem "normal," but some sounds perceived by the child are distorted. For instance, the ability to distinguish between different consonants may be impaired, which leads to problems with reading and language.

The children most adversely affected by the triad of otitis media, hearing loss, and delayed development are those living in low socioeconomic conditions (although the effects are by no means restricted to these children). This includes the growing number of children living with a single parent and those of immigrant parents. In both groups, the financial resources, access to good health care, availability of nuitritious food and nutrition information is severely restricted. In immigrant populations, parents are often uneducated about the need to treat otitis media and the consequences that may follow if hearing loss is persistent.

Sadly, many children with hearing impairment are labeled early in life as learning disabled or unintelligent, much like "deaf" persons were labeled in the past. Proper treatment and monitoring of young children with middle ear effusion is important if we are to effectively address their needs. The underlying factors leading up to otitis media must also be addressed. These are discussed in the following chapter.

Chapter 5

Causes of Childhood Ear Infections

By definition, otitis media is a disease of the ears. Fluid accumulates in the middle ear, pressure develops in the middle ear, bacteria invade the middle ear, and pain occurs in the middle ear. Quite naturally then, doctors should directly treat the ears with whatever means are possible. Or should they? One great weaknesses in modern medical practice is the compartmentalization of the body. This means that when a problem arises in a body structure, the problem is perceived to reside only there. It is believed to be in no way related to events that occur elsewhere in the body. However, this view is rapidly being shown to be erroneous.

Consider that, for many decades and to this day, holistic doctors have contended that stress, emotions, and the mind have a direct and profound effect on susceptibility to illness. Failure to address these factors has led to continued susceptibility to illness. The allopathic* response to this thinking was:

Allopathic refers to the use of therapies that produce effects that differ from the disease being treated. The term is usually associated with modern medical practice and refers to the use of drugs, surgery, chemotherapy, and radiation. Compare this with *homeopathic* (discussed later), which is based on the use of minute quantities of substances that in massive doses produce effects similar to those of the disease being treated.[1]

The mind and body are in no way related. This position was published in medical journals as recently as 1985. Yet within the past few years a new field of study called psychoneuroimmunology has emerged. Researchers in this field, based at major universities around the world, are now documenting the vital link between the mind and the immune system.

Holistic doctors counsel their patients on the need for whole grains, fruits and vegetables, and the need to restrict the intake of processed foods. They often prescribe vitamins as well. This practice has also been met with scorn from allopathic doctors. Their reasoning: refined foods do not contribute to ill health because they're fortified with vitamins and minerals. The taking of vitamin supplements only leads to "expensive urine."

Yet today, we've learned from sophisticated research worldwide that food processing contributes to substantial loss of nutrients, which is not replaced through fortification. Moreover, we now know of more than 120 diseases in which the genetic requirement for certain nutrients may be 10 to 100 times the average. Nutrient supplementation is essential in order for such people to lead normal lives. Finally, no one can argue with the fact that the enzymes needed to drive every metabolic process in the human body are completely dependent upon the vitamins and trace minerals we provide through our diet.[2]

The evidence documenting the interconnectedness of *all* body parts and functions is accumulating at a breathtaking pace. As our understanding grows, it is clear that viewing any illness as a localized problem is not sufficient. Doctors who treat otitis media as though it is simply a middle ear problem fail to recognize this interconnectedness and frequently overlook the factors that initially give rise to otitis media. Otitis media is an inflammation of the middle ear. All the events that occur in the middle ear—swelling, pain, infection, complications—are important and must be addressed. However, these events may only be the sequel to events that occur elsewhere in the body.

The cause of otitis media is not fully understood. There may, in fact, be no singular cause of the disease. What probably occurs is a multiplicity of events that interact to take advantage of lowered immune function, underdeveloped eustachian tube muscles, respiratory congestion, excessive mucus production, nutritional inadequacy, or any number of other factors. In this section, I present a synthesis of the major contributing factors in middle ear infection. In each case, prevention and treatment solutions are available that take advantage of our understanding of the causes presented here.

The four main causes of otitis media are:*

- Allergy.
- Infection.
- Mechanical Obstruction.
- Nutritional Deficiency.

Allergy

Allergy is called the great masquerader because it can contribute to and mimic many illnesses with which we don't usually associate allergy.[4] From recurrent colds to bronchitis, bedwetting to headaches, enlarged tonsils to diarrhea, allergy can play a significant role. To children with recurrent middle ear infection, allergy is indeed the "great masquerader." Allergy can contribute to swollen tonsils, nasal and sinus congestion, swollen mucous membranes of the eustachian tube, and ultimately, fluid in the middle ear. In some children, the persistence of

---

*In 1976, W. Leonard Draper, M.D. stated that childhood otitis media has multiple causes, and multiple phases. He listed among the causes allergy, infection, and mechanical blockage. Since 1976, our understanding of nutrition has expanded substantially making it clear that nutritional factors also play an important role in the development of otitis media.[3]

allergy leads to the chronic buildup of a very viscous and mucoid fluid in the middle ear.

Not all children with allergies develop middle ear problems, and not all children with middle ear problems have them because of allergies. But in children whose earaches are due to allergy, neglecting to treat the allergy (or the underlying factors that lead to the development of allergies) often results in recurrent infections.

Evidence demonstrating the role of allergy in middle ear problems has been steadily accumulating over the past four decades. A study of 540 children by W. Leonard Draper, M.D., showed that secretory otitis media was more than twice as frequent in allergic children than in non-allergic children.[5] Draper also noted, in a study of 100 allergic children, that approximately 50 percent had fluid in the ears.[6] Poor eustachian tube function—believed to be one of the prime factors leading to the development of middle ear infection—has been found to occur in almost one-third of allergic children.[7]

No one is certain of the percentage of children with allergy-related otitis media. The available evidence suggests that from 11 to 85 percent of cases have an allergic component.[8, 9] Dr. L.Q. Pang, Clinical Professor of Surgery at the University of Hawaii Medical School, insists that allergy plays a significant role in otitis media. He states that "a large percentage of chronic suppurative otitis media with a central perforation [of the eardrum] is due to an allergy."[10]

Dr. D.C. Heiner and his associates report in the *Annals of Allergy* that "childhood otitis media may be solely, or partially due to food allergy." He goes on to stress that much of the tonsilar or adenoid swelling, and even upper airway obstruction, may be caused or aggravated by food allergies.[11] Doris Rapp, M.D., author of numerous books on childhood allergy, states that avoidance of the major offending food items, or indoor problematic allergens, can help many patients with otitis media. More importantly, she says that "by eliminating the cause of the medical problem [through allergy management], it is often possible to obviate [eliminate] not only the need for surgery, but also the necessity to mask the patient's symptoms with medications."[12]

Dr. George Shambaugh, Professor Emeritus of Otolaryngology at Northwestern University and former president of the American Academy of Otolaryngology, gave an address in 1982 entitled, "Serous Otitis: Are Tubes the Answer?" In his lecture, he addresses the question of allergy, stating, "Although allergies in children are often hard to identify by the usual allergy scratch tests, I've found that a program of allergic management with attention to hidden or delayed-in-onset food allergy helps me manage recurrent ear problems in children. Moreover, my results with allergy management are far better than those obtained by putting children on prolonged courses of antibiotics, and relying on tubes to clear up the condition."[13]

If allergies are a factor in middle ear infection, there should be evidence that shows a capacity for allergens to cause adverse changes in the middle ear and eustachian tube. We also would expect children with allergy-related earaches to improve with some form of allergy management.

Allergens can cause direct changes within the middle ear and eustachian tube. Dr. Robert O'Conner and his colleagues have observed that significant and rapid pressure changes take place in the middle ear of children when their nasal passages are exposed to allergens.[14] Other scientists have found that allergens can cause obstruction of the eustachian tube that lasts for up to 14 days. Often, a blocked eustachian tube can be encouraged to open by swallowing, but in cases where tube blockage occurs because of allergy, swallowing appears to have little impact. These findings suggest an allergic basis for eustachian tube obstruction and possibly for the development of middle ear disease.[15]

The response of allergic children with otitis media to proper allergy management can be swift and dramatic. Dr. John P. McGovern and his associates studied 512 children with allergy and middle ear problems. Using careful allergy management, these doctors reported good or excellent results with 97 percent of the children.[16] A 1982 report in the *International Journal of Pediatric Otorhinolaryngology* revealed that elimination diets—for children who tested positive for foods—were useful in the treatment of otitis media. A significant finding in this study of 67 children was that "fewer operations were needed in the treatment of patients with elimination diets."[17]

Consider the case of Chris. Chris first became a patient of mine at age two. His chief symptom was impetigo, which is a highly contagious infection of the skin. Chris had pustules on his face and hands. Whenever his face began to heal, he reinfected it with his hands. Chris had been treated at a local university hospital with a variety of drugs, including antibiotics. The impetigo did not respond to any therapy. When I examined Chris, I first looked at his diet and nutritional status. He was hooked on bread, rolls, cereals, crackers and anything that contained grains. This suggested food allergy. The balance of his diet consisted of dairy products. Following elimination testing, it was clear that Chris was sensitive to gluten and dairy products. (Gluten is a very sticky protein found in wheat, rye, oats, and barley.) After beginning a new diet that eliminated foods containing gluten and dairy, Chris' impetigo began to improve significantly, only to return when an enthusiastic grandmother fed Chris some cookies (which contained gluten). One week following his grandmother's "gluten challenge," the impetigo again improved. However, it did not heal completely, suggesting that something else was amiss.

Many of his initial signs of nutritional deficiency improved following the dietary changes, but it was evident that he still suffered from zinc and fatty acid deficiency. I placed him on supplements of zinc and fatty acids. Following this, the remnants of impetigo that remained resolved fully. Chris had very few problems until about age five, when he developed a problem with recurrent otitis media. Chris was brought to me after six months of recurrent earaches. When I examined him, he showed signs of food allergy. Over the years, Chris was able to rotate (see chapter 6 for a discussion of rotation diets) the offending foods back into his diet without adverse consequences. Upon questioning his parents, I learned that Chris was being given yogurt almost daily. His parents believed yogurt was acceptable because it was a cultured dairy product. In Chris' case, it wasn't. Within weeks of removing the yogurt from Chris' diet, his earaches cleared up.

There are a substantial number of children who continue to have middle ear fluid despite repeated antibiotic therapy. In many cases (up to 75 percent),[18] the fluid contains no bacteria. In instances such as this, doctors frequently resort to surgery (adenoidectomy, tonsillectomy, myringotomy or tubes) in an effort to clear up the fluid in the middle ear. In children in whom allergy is a principal contributor, we would expect middle ear fluid to remain, since these surgeries are not designed to eliminate the source of the fluid. In 1982, Dr. K. Ojala addressed this issue in an extensive study of the allergic cells in the middle ear fluid of children who continued to have fluid despite surgical treatment. He compared these children with children who had postsurgical dry ears or normal ears. At the completion of his study, Dr. Ojala concluded, "It would seem that atopy [allergy] is probably one cause of persistent therapy-resistant otitis media, and it must be taken into account when considering treatment of a chronic ear."[19]

In another study, 92 children with otitis media who had been treated unsuccessfully with tubes were tested for allergic sensitivity. Of the 85 that were treated with hyposensitization (which is only one form of allergic management), 57 were able to have their tubes removed with no fluid recurrence.[20]

Besides having direct effects on the middle ear, there is evidence that allergens, especially food allergens, can cause immune system suppression, which limits the ability of the body to fight infection. Food allergies are often the result of intestinal problems. Intestinal problems are a common source of illness among children. According to Russell M. Jaffe, M.D., Ph.D., of the National Institutes of Health, if intestinal integrity is low, due to excessive antibiotic use, malabsorption, high intake of refined food, or other factors, fragments of poorly digested food are often absorbed intact. These partially digested proteins are known as IBPs (Incomplete Breakdown Products). When IBPs are absorbed into the bloodstream, the child's immune system recognizes them as foreign (because the immune system is unaccustomed to seeing large protein fragments). The white blood cells then mount an attack as though the IBPs were hazardous invaders.

Dr. Jaffe has shown that when the blood levels of IBPs are high, the ability of white blood cells to engulf and destroy bacteria falls to as low as two per three-hour period, compared to the normal rate of over 50 during the same period. The total number of lymphocytes circulating in the bloodstream at any given time is somewhat limited. Dr. Jaffe states that if we tie up our lymphocytes in mounting an attack against this circulating food residue, we reduce the number of lymphocytes available to fight infection.[21] Thus, allergy appears to have both a direct and indirect adverse effect on a child's ability to fight infection in the middle ear.

What is an Allergy?

Doctors disagree on the extent to which allergies play a role in middle ear problems. Many allergists contend that what people call allergies today are not really allergies. They argue that "true" allergy requires an IgE reaction. IgE stands for immunoglobulin E, which is a protein commonly produced by white blood cells during allergic reactions. Much contemporary research shows that the body reacts adversely to foreign substances in a variety of ways—not only through IgE. In fact, IgE reactions play a role in the earaches of perhaps only 15 percent of children described as allergic on the basis of clinical and laboratory evidence.[22] Dr. E. Pastorello has found a surprisingly high incidence of food intolerance that is not related to IgE.[23]

To speak accurately of the way in which people adversely react to substances with which they come in contact, we have to use the terms allergy and hypersensitivity. *Allergy* is defined as an adverse response brought about by exposure to a substance in the environment—called an allergen. These reactions occur because the immune system recognizes the substance(s) as a threat and goes into an attack mode to eliminate the threat. *Hypersensitivity* (the term intolerance is sometimes used) is an adverse reaction to a substance for any other reason.

Figure 2 **Research Linking Ear Infection to Allergy**		
Researcher/Journal	**Year**	**Allergy Type**
Draper, *Clinical Ecology*	1976	Food-Airborne
Shambaugh, American Academy of Otolaryngology (Lecture)	1982	Food-Airborne
Mogi, *Acta Otorhinolaryngology Belgium*	1983	Food-Airborne
Friedman, *Journal of Allergy and Clinical Immunology*	1983	Food-Airborne
Bernstein, *American Journal of Otolaryngology*	1983	Airborne
Rapp, *American Journal of Otolaryngology*	1984	Food-Airborne
Heiner, *Annals of Allergy*	1984	Food-Airborne
Kraemer, *Clinical Reviews in Allergy*	1984	Airborne
Ackerman, *Journal of Allergy and Clinical Immunology*	1984	Airborne
O'Conner, *Annals of Allergy*	1985	Airborne
Asman, *International Pediatrics*	1988	Food-Airborne

An example of true allergy is a child who develops a runny nose, watery eyes, sneezing, and stuffiness when exposed to ragweed pollen. When the blood is tested in such children, IgE antibodies are often elevated, along with an elevation in the white cells called eosinophils. Examples of hypersensitivity include adverse reactions to two common food additives— monosodium glutamate (MSG) and sulfites. MSG—a substance to which many people are sensitive—is used widely as a flavor enhancer. Sulfites are a family of compounds used to preserve the whiteness of foods such as sugar, flour, baking powder, and dried fruit.

Hypersensitivity reactions to foods or additives are frequently due to nutritional deficiency or problems with improperly functioning enzymes. For example, scientists have observed that many MSG-sensitive individuals who are given B6 are no longer sensitive to MSG.[24] This suggests that the enzyme needed to properly metabolize MSG is enhanced by B6. In individuals who are not B6-supplemented, ingested MSG builds up in the system rather than being processed and eliminated efficiently.

The enzyme that helps to break down excess sulfite happens to be dependent upon the micro-trace element molybdenum.[25] Deficiency of molybdenum can impair the enzyme, which leads to a build-up of sulfite in the body, which leads to symptoms. The symptoms persist until either the sulfites are eliminated from the diet, or molybdenum is added to the diet. Sulfites can aggravate or cause upper respiratory reactions in sensitive individuals. I've even observed cases of sulfite-related otitis media.

How Allergies May Contribute to Middle Ear Problems

- Allergens may trigger collapse or narrowing of the eustachian tube. This interferes with normal opening and closing, thereby reducing ventilation of the middle ear.

- Allergens may cause swollen tonsils or adenoids, leading to reduced elimination (or drainage) of lymph fluid (see Heiner). This mechanically obstructs the eustachian tube opening.

- Allergens can initiate excessive production of mucus and serous fluid. This results in reduced ventilation of the middle ear, reduced drainage of the middle ear, and slowed movement of white blood cells to the site of infection.

- Allergens, especially food allergens, can inhibit the white blood cells' ability to digest and destroy bacteria. (See Jaffe.)

This is a fairly simple assessment of the way in which allergy contributes to middle ear problems. The true mechanism is not well understood, and at this time, is considered theoretical.

The Most Common Offenders

Allergy and hypersensitivity reactions can be triggered by virtually any substance to which a child is exposed. There are two major categories of substances which initiate these reactions— food and airborne. Within these categories, there are some substances that contribute to otitis media more frequently than others. This reduces the pursuit of potential offenders from thousands to only a handful. In general, food allergy/hypersensitivity contributes more to otitis media than does airborne. However, each category contains important offenders.

Food Allergy and Hypersensitivity

In a study of 1,000 patients with food allergy, Dr. Frederic Speer found that milk, chocolate, cola, corn, citrus, and egg were the most common allergens. Milk allergies were especially common in children under two.[26] Of all foods, cow's milk and other dairy products are probably the number one contributor to childhood ear problems. These and other common allergens implicated in otitis media are listed below.

- Dairy products, including milk, butter, cheese, yogurt, cottage cheese, cow's milk formula, and *ice cream*.

- Wheat, including not only bread and cereal, but anything that contains wheat such as gravies, crackers, and cookies.

- Eggs or anything containing eggs.

- Chocolate.

- Citrus, especially oranges and orange juice.

- Corn, or anything containing corn, such as corn flakes.

- Soy. This is especially a problem with infant formula. Dr. William Crook states that 25 percent of infants with a milk allergy develop an allergy to soy.

- Peanuts and other nuts. Peanut butter is a great favorite among children and a frequent contributor to childhood health problems.

- Shellfish.

- Sugar.

- Yeast.

Food allergy can be a nemesis because the offenders hide among a variety of foods children consume every day. In many cases, the foods to which a child is allergic or sensitive are those that she eats the most. Commonly, children are addicted to foods. The cravings can be so intense that a child will refuse to eat unless her "favorite" food is given at mealtime. I've seen this occur with cheese, crackers, milk, peanut butter, and virtually all items on the above list.

Foods that are consumed every day, or several times a day, can lead to the development of allergy or hypersensitivity to that food. Children with a daily diet that consists of only a handful of items are at risk to developing food allergies. I'm reminded of a patient who developed severe inflammatory arthritis every July and August. This summertime flare-up of symptoms had been a mystery to her doctors for many years. When I asked about any dietary changes that might occur during this time of year, she said, "I love tomatoes. When I'm able to get them fresh from the garden, I eat as many as I can." This woman consumed tomatoes on occasion during the year with no ill effects. However, when summertime harvest yielded a bounty of her favorite food, she consumed tomatoes several times a day, almost every day. This level of consumption overloaded her system and triggered an inflammatory response. This is a dramatic illustration of the way in which overconsumption, or frequent consumption of a food, can lead to problems that might not occur with the same food under ordinary circumstances.

In chapter 2, I described how antibiotic use contributes to the development of food allergies by eradicating beneficial intestinal bacteria. In one study, *all* children suffering from symptoms of food allergies had evidence of deficiencies of *Lactobacilli* and *Bifidobacteria* in the intestinal tract. They also had an overgrowth of other enteric bacteria.[27] When the intestinal bacteria are restored through supplementation, food allergies frequently improve. (See chapter 6.)

Airborne Allergy and Sensitivity

Airborne substances easily contribute to upper respiratory and ear problems because they are in constant contact with the mucous membranes of these parts of the body. In children who are not allergic, airborne allergens usually don't cause much trouble (although one family of indoor air pollutants, discussed later, can cause significant mucous membrane irritation even in non-allergic children).

The average adult spends only one hour per day outdoors. The average child spends only slightly more time outdoors, especially in northern climates. Because the vast *quantity* of air children breath is indoor air, it is essential that the indoor air be of good *quality*. Unfortunately, the indoor air in most American homes, schools, and offices is full of contaminants. These pollutants are contributing to an increase in chronic health complaints in both children and adults. The most common indoor air pollutants are:

- Cigarette smoke.
- Volatile organic compounds.
- Pollen.
- Carbon monoxide.
- Animal dander.
- House dust.
- Mold.
- Fungi.
- Sulfur dioxide.
- Bacteria.

The most pernicious airborne irritant in otitis media is sidestream **cigarette smoke**. Dr. Michael Kraemer and his colleagues reported in the *Journal of the American Medical Association* in 1983 that the incidence of otitis media with effusion increases nearly three-fold when a child is exposed to two or more household smokers. When exposed to smoke from more than three packs of cigarettes per day, the risk increases four-fold.[28]

Children of smoking parents are admitted to hospitals nearly 28 percent more often than children of non-smoking parents. Those exposed to second-hand cigarette smoke also lose more days to sickness from respiratory ailments (which is significant because 50 percent of all earaches follow an upper respiratory problem of some type).[29] See Figure 3.

There are probably many reasons why cigarette smoke causes an increase in childhood ear infections. Recent evidence suggests that the level of vitamin E is lower in the lungs of smokers than in the lungs of nonsmokers. Vitamin E is an important antioxidant nutrient that protects cell membranes from free-radical damage. Free radicals are highly reactive chemical species that cause destruction of cells through chain reactions. Scientists estimate that one puff of sidestream (second-hand) cigarette smoke contains up to one hundred-trillion or 100,000,000,000,000 (10^{14}) free radicals.[31] When the delicate lining of the respiratory tract is exposed to the large number of free radicals found in cigarette smoke (see Figure 4), significant demands are placed on the antioxidant defense mechanism of the respiratory tract, leading to vitamin E deficiency.

Figure 3 Comparative "Sick Days" Among Children of Smoking and Nonsmoking Households		
	Children's Restricted Activity Days	**Children's Bed-Disability Days**
No Smokers in Home (control)	—	—
1 Smoker in Home	+ 7 percent	+ 14 percent
2 or More Smokers in Home	+ 29 percent	+ 29 percent
45 or More Cigarettes Per Day	+ 46 percent	+ 43 percent
(Adapted from Bonham and Wilson, 1981)[30]		

Vitamin C is another member of the antioxidant defense system designed to protect the delicate lining of our cell membranes from injury. Cigarette smoke causes vitamin C to be excreted more rapidly in the urine of smokers and presumably in the urine of children exposed to second-hand smoke as well.

The depletion of protective antioxidant nutrients by exposure to smoke is significant since sidestream smoke is often

Figure 4
Principal Constituents of Cigarette Smoke*

Particles:

tar	pyrene
nicotine	benzo (a) pyrene
perylene	benzo (e) pyrene
benzo (ghi) perylene	dibenz(a,j)anthracene
fluoranthene	dibenz(ah)anthracene,
benzo(a)fluorene	ideno (2,3-ed) chrysene,
benzo(b)fluorene	benz(a)anthracene
cadmium	anthanthrene
phenol	benzo(b/k/j)fluoranthrene

Gases and Vapors:

water	acrolein
carbon monoxide	formaldehyde
ammonia	toluene
carbon dioxide	acetone
nitrogen oxides	polonium-210
hydrogen cyanide	

Source: U.S. National Research Council, Committee on Indoor Pollutants, 1981, p. IV-101.[32]

*Many airborne pollutants are absorbed as freely, or more freely through the lungs than through the intestines or skin. Therefore, breathing some of these substances is not much different from eating or drinking them.

more toxic than inhaled smoke (especially when filtered cigarettes are used). The reduced antioxidant levels result in changes in the cells lining the respiratory tract, leading to a reduced ability to remove allergens, bacteria, and viruses. The lining of the middle ear cavity consists of cells very similar to those lining the lungs and other parts of the respiratory tract. The irritants found in smoke cause much the same damage to the lining of the middle ear as they do to the lungs and nasal passages.

Sidestream smoke has been shown to paralyze cilia within the respiratory tract. The lining of the middle ear and respiratory tract consists of a layer of stratified, column-shaped cells covered with tiny hairlike cilia that help remove allergens and microbes from the middle ear. During exposure to cigarette smoke, the cilia are destroyed or impaired. This reduces the ability of the middle ear to remove invading microbes and allergens. The consequences include middle ear effusion and infection.

House dust is another common airborne offender that can contribute to otitis media. It contributes to illness because of its ability to carry tremendous numbers of allergens, toxicants, and microbes. House dust is a complex mixture of hundreds of items including lint, snips of hair, oils, animal dander (including human skin), and particles of textiles from rugs, bedding, furniture, drapes, carpet padding, clothing, and pillows. One teaspoon of house dust can contain from 5 to 10 million microbes—including some very nasty bacteria and viruses. After a short incubation period, the numbers can rise into the billions.

One of the most common irritants found in household dust is the house dust mite. According to G.W. Wharton, many people are more allergic to mites than to other house dust components.[33] This tiny arthropod feeds on human skin and resides in mattresses, carpeting, draperies, and any household item that harbors dust. Vacuum cleaners left standing with a partially full bag often serve as hotels in which millions of house dust mites eat, reproduce, live, and grow old.

House dust is also a principal source of lead, cadmium, and other heavy metals. In studies of cognitive function in children, Dr. Robert Thatcher and his associates showed that serum and tissue lead and cadmium levels in children correlated directly with the level of house dust. Apparently, the children come in contact with heavy metals through the dust that collects on their hands during play. The dust is then transferred to mouth by normal hand-to-mouth activity. In these studies, lead and cadmium were shown to have direct adverse effect on verbal IQ and performance IQ.[34] Lead and cadmium are also known to have an adverse effect on immune function. Reduction of house dust is one important element in controlling exposure to these metals. (Incidentally, children with adequate levels of zinc appear to be insulated against the adverse effects of cadmium, while those with adequate calcium are insulated against the adverse effects of lead.)

In the average home, roughly 40 pounds of house dust are produced annually. It is a significant problem for infants and toddlers because they spend the better part of their day crawling and shuffling around on the floor. Dust is further circulated by common forced-air furnaces and vacuum cleaners. (See chapter 7 on prevention.) To the allergic child, the continual dose of allergens and microbes in house dust creates significant upper respiratory irritation and contributes to chronic upper respiratory disease, otitis media, tonsillitis, and rhinitis. Children who are not "allergic" may still suffer, due to the presence of such large numbers of agents that can potentially challenge the immune system.

A fairly recent addition to the family of indoor air pollutants/respiratory irritants is a group of chemicals called **volatile organic compounds** (VOC). VOC are organic chemicals that evaporate at temperatures of 32 degrees Fahrenheit and higher. They are constituents of common household items. Among these are cleaning compounds, newsprint, mothballs, and even furniture. Building materials are one of the greatest sources of VOC. These include particle board, paint, varnish, caulking compounds, carpeting, vinyl floor covering, and more.

We are only beginning to understand the scope of this problem. In 1985, the EPA studied 11 VOCs indoors. Their findings revealed unacceptable levels of compounds such as benzene, trichloroethane, and styrene—all of which are not only membrane irritants but carcinogens as well. Levels of all tested compounds were higher indoors than outdoors. The home's age or location seemed to have no bearing on pollutant levels. From new urban homes to old rural homes, the problem of volatile pollutants was similar.[35]

In Baton Rouge, Houston, and Greensborough, the EPA measured levels of 32 volatile chemicals and found all to be higher in the indoor air than in the outdoor air.[36] Public access buildings such as schools, office buildings, and day care facilities are often among the worst offenders. In a Washington, D.C., home for the elderly, 350 different volatile chemicals were identified *in the air*. Of these, 35 were found at all locations tested, and 12 were known carcinogens or mutagens.[37]

The air quality in homes is also among the worst. In Oak Ridge, Tennessee, federal scientists monitored 40 homes for the presence of organic vapors in the air. During the study period, they identified between 20 and 150 solvents and other volatile chemicals in the indoor air of *each structure*! Only 10 were found in the outdoor air.[38] These and similar studies reveal that indoor air pollution is a serious and growing problem.

Where Do Indoor Air Pollutants Come From?

Indoor air pollutants are generated from building materials and household products. Almost every aspect of our lives involves the use of synthetic materials. These synthetic materials release vapors that, over time, contribute to ill health in a large number of people.

Carpeting is one of the worst offenders. Carpeting is comprised of synthetic fibers derived from petroleum. At various stages of processing, chemicals are added to carpet to make it stain-resistant and fire-resistant. Insecticides and fungicides are often added to carpeting to protect it against mold, mildew, and fungus. These chemicals are highly toxic and highly irritating. What's worse, their vapors are released from the carpeting as the carpet ages. The "new carpet" smell is actually a chemical soup that wafts its way through the air. When carpeting is cleaned by professional cleaning services, more toxic compounds are added. Naptha, a known carcinogen, is often used in the cleaning process. In addition, insecticides and stain-

Figure 5
Summary of Other Studies of Indoor Air Pollutants

Molhave	Found elevated levels of benzene & toluene in 39 dwellings.
Jarke	Found increased concentration of organics in 34 Chicago homes.
Leberet	Concluded that 35 of 35 organics had mean indoor levels greater than outdoor levels in 134 tested homes. Seven of these indoor levels exceeded outdoor levels by 10 times. Tobacco smoking was correlated with increase of 10 organics.
Seifert	Measured 15 homes in Berlin; all had increased levels of toluene(*) and xylene from printed material.
Gammage	Detected gasoline vapors in 40 Tennessee homes, most with attached garages.

39, 40, 41, 42, 43

Note: Many early monitoring studies of indoor pollutants have been done in Europe. Those conducted in American homes yield similar results. Presently, European governments have taken the lead in reducing the indoor contaminants in the home. The U.S. government has made little progress in this regard, evidenced by the relaxed standards regarding formaldehyde in building materials.

(*) Toluene, a solvent that is a carcinogen and well-known mucous membrane irritant, is the most common airborne pollutant isolated in all studies.

proofing agents are applied during the cleaning.

Formaldehyde is a familiar indoor air pollutant. It is found in everything from cosmetics to clothing. One of the richest sources of formaldehyde is the waferboard used in the walls and subflooring of almost all new homes.

Old newspapers stored indoors can outgas toxic vapors for months. The printing ink contains a complex mixture of chemicals including toluene and xylene. Fuel used for heating can cause problems as well. Children in homes where wood stoves are used suffer from more respiratory ailments than children in homes where wood stoves are not used.[44] The list of sources of volatile pollutants is almost endless.

How Volatile Indoor Air Pollutants Contribute to Ear Infections

Most cases of otitis media with effusion share a common characteristic—inflammation of the mucous membrane of the middle ear and/or eustachian tube. Moreover, otitis media is frequently preceded by inflammation of the upper respiratory tract. These delicate tissues, while possessing some form of protection, are susceptible to the continuous presence of irritants in the air.

As discussed above, the vapors often found in indoor air are common constituents of the building materials used in the construction of homes, offices, and schools. When the vapors of building materials were analyzed, it was found that as high as *80 percent were known mucous membrane irritants*.[46] In other words, the items used to build and furnish our homes, schools, day care centers, and offices are replete with invisible, often odorless gases that can initiate inflammation of the middle ear (also eyes, nose, throat, and lungs). At first, constant exposure to even low levels of these airborne gases overwhelms the antioxidant defense system. As exposure continues, inflammatory and immune changes occur that can contribute to ongoing respiratory and middle ear complaints.

This category of indoor air pollutants has become serious only since the mid-1970s, because of the increase in tighter, energy-efficient homes, coupled with a rapid increase in the use of synthetic materials. Ironically, the incidence of otitis media has increased dramatically during the same period. While it is difficult to prove a link between indoor air pollutants and

Figure 6
Examples of Organic Compound Types and Potential Indoor Sources

Pollutant Type	Example	Indoor Sources
Aliphatic hydrocarbons	Propane, butane, hexane, limonene	Cooking and heating fuels, aerosol propellants, cleaning compounds, refrigerants, lubricants, flavoring agents, perfume base
Halogenated hydrocarbons	Methyl chloroform, methylene chloride, PCBs	Aerosol propellants, fumigants, pesticides, refrigerants, and degreasing, dewaxing, and dry cleaning solvents
Aromatic hydrocarbons	Benzene, toluene, xylenes	Paints, varnishes, glues, enamels, lacquers, cleaners
Alcohols	Ethanol, methanol	Window cleaners, paint thinners, cosmetics, adhesives, human breath
Ketones	Acetone	Lacquers, varnishes, polish removers, adhesives
Aldehydes	Formaldehyde, nonanal	Fungicides, germicides, disinfectants, artificial and permanent-press textiles, paper, particle boards, cosmetics, flavoring agents, etc.

From *Indoor Air and Human Health*, by R.B. Gammage and S.V. Kaye. Copyright 1985, Lewis Publishers, Inc., Chelsea, MI, p. 391. Used with permission.[45]

otitis media, it is very likely that these volatile pollutants have contributed to some of the upper respiratory irritation that often creates susceptibility to middle ear problems. The constant presence of airborne irritants also may impede the recovery of middle ear problems due to other causes.

Outdoor air pollution may be contributing indirectly to an increase in otitis media. Recently, Dr. Philip Landrigan of the American Academy of Pediatrics reported to the United States Congress that the incidence of childhood asthma cases has increased 25 percent from 1982 to 1986. In 1987, more than 760,000 children were hospitalized with a respiratory disease. Upper respiratory infection, lung congestion, and nasal congestion have long been considered risk factors to otitis media. Dr. Landrigan says that the problem of poor air quality has gotten worse in many of the 90 cities that violate the Clean Air Act of 1970.[47]

*   *   *

According to a 1983 report in the *British Medical Journal*, the incidence of allergy in children under five more than doubled from 1970 to 1982.[48] During this period, the incidence of otitis media has more than doubled as well. The reasons behind this dramatic increase are a source of ongoing speculation and research. One might suggest that there is a relationship between the increase in allergy and the increase in otitis media. Based on the available evidence, allergy and hypersensitivity to either food or airborne substances deserves consideration in the child with recurrent otitis media.

Infection

Under certain conditions, bacteria present in the upper respiratory tract find their way up the eustachian tube into the middle ear. Once in the middle ear chamber, they contribute to the damaging events with which we usually associate infection. When middle ear fluid is cultured for bacteria, the most common bacteria found are *Haemophilus influenzae* and *Streptococcus pneumoniae*. These are called *pathogenic* organisms, which refers to their ability to produce disease. Cases of otitis media in which *S. pneumoniae* is involved tend to occur with severe pain and fever, while those associated with *H. influenzae* have less pain and fever, but more commonly affect both ears.[49, 50]

In a report of bacteria found in middle ear fluid from a total of 3,583 children from three countries, Dr. J.O. Klein observed the presence of either *S. pneumoniae* (35 percent) or *H. influenzae* (20 percent) in a total of 55 percent of cases.[51] During a period from 1980 to 1985, other investigators found that *S. pneumoniae* and *H. influenzae* comprised 50.7 percent of bacteria isolated from the middle ear fluid of their patients (29.8 and 20.9 percent respectively).[52]

Other bacteria have been found in middle ear fluid as well. However, most of these are normal residents of the body. Doctors disagree about whether these "indigenous" bacteria contribute in any way to middle ear problems. Viruses—which are believed to contribute to a substantial percentage of childhood upper respiratory complaints—are only rarely found in middle ear fluid.[53] However, chronic viral infections may contribute to immune suppression.

The identification of bacteria in middle ear fluid is useful but fails to provide an answer to one important question. Do these bacteria cause otitis media, or are they merely opportunists taking advantage of a weakened child or hospitable middle ear environment? Without this discussion of child susceptibility, there can be no realistic discussion of infection. The problem with the contemporary western concept of infection is that doctors often overlook the question of susceptibility.

Efforts to demonstrate the importance of host susceptibility have, on occasion, taken on dramatic proportion. The great Russian pathologist Eli Metchnikoff once drank a solution containing millions of cholera bacteria to prove that a healthy individual would not contract the disease and die. Metchnikoff experienced only mild diarrhea as a result of this experiment.

Figure 7				
Types of Bacteria Found in Middle Ear Fluid				
	Percentage			
Bacteria	**1**	**2**	**3**	**4**
S. pneumoniae	29.8	35		33
H. influenzae	20	20.9		23
Streptococcus, g A	8	—		2
B. catarrhalis	11.7	3		
Staph aureus	2	1.6		
S. pyogenes	3.1	—		
Gram negative enteric bacteria	1	—		
Mixed organisms	2	19.1		7
None or non-pathogenic	29	19.6	42	33

1—Klein, et al, 1980 (3,583 subjects)[54]
2—Asman, Fireman, 1988 (1,432 subjects)[55]
3—Pelton, et al, 1980 (122 subjects)[56]
4—Schwartz, et al, 1978[57]

Differences in the above findings may be due, in part, to the way in which the investigators classified non-pathogenic organisms.

As predicted, he did not contract cholera.

Nutritional status has long been associated with susceptibility to disease. Children suffering from generalized malnutrition are known to suffer from impaired immune function and are at increased risk of succumbing to infections of all types.[58] Overall malnutrition is not even required. Recent studies in the U.S. and Scandinavia have shown that deficiency of only one or two trace elements can render a child more susceptible to infection.[59] Zinc deficiency can cause the thymus gland to shrink substantially, thereby inhibiting cell-mediated immunity.[60] When diets are low in essential fatty acids, other lymphoid tissue atrophies, resulting in depressed immunity. Folic acid is among the most commonly deficient of all nutrients. Lack of this vitamin can lead to reduced resistance to infection.[61] Deficiency of any of the following nutrients has thus far been shown to increase susceptibility to infection: folic acid, pantothenic acid, pyridoxine, riboflavin, vitamin A, vitamin C, vitamin E, copper, iron, magnesium, and zinc.[62]

Lowered immune function, and therefore susceptibility to infection, can be due to genetic factors. Remarkably, it also may be due to the nutritional intake of a parent or grandparent. Evidence for this finding was supplied in a now-famous animal study by Dr. Lucille Hurley, who showed that when a pregnant mother's zinc status is low, the offspring show signs of immune deficiency. This immune insufficiency can persist for up to three generations. The findings are especially significant because the immune problems can often be passed from generation to generation in spite of supplementation with zinc.[63]

Even consumption of sugar can lower immune function by reducing the ability of white blood cells to digest and destroy bacteria. The lowered immune effect can last for five hours or more following the ingestion of sugar.[64] Children with low numbers of intestinal *Lactobacilli* and *Bifidobacteria* are more likely to succumb to infection than are children who harbor optimum levels of these microbes in their intestinal tract.

Environmental factors common today also lower resistance to infection. Cadmium toxicity has been shown to reduce resistance to both bacterial and viral infection. Cadmium is a contaminant of the food, air, and water in various areas of the country. It is also found in second-hand cigarette smoke. Lead also inhibits immunity. Lead is found in leaded paint and canned food, and is a major constituent of house dust in some areas. The adverse effects of both cadmium and lead on children are significant. Not only do these metals cause direct adverse effects on immunity, but they also deplete the body of zinc and calcium, respectively.

Unfortunately, many doctors have ignored the rapidly emerging data that point to altered nutritional status as a significant contributor to susceptibility to infection. They have chosen instead to rely on their arsenal of antibiotics to combat invading organisms that, given the needed raw materials, the child's immune system might defeat alone.

If infection were indeed the *cause* of otitis media, one would suspect that antibiotics would be successful in treating the disease—provided the right antibiotic is given. However, many children with otitis media do not respond to antibiotics. In a study by Dr. David Teele and his colleagues, 57 percent of children who did not respond to antibiotic therapy had sterile middle ear fluid 36 hours after therapy was begun,[65] meaning the bacteria had been eradicated. Yet middle ear fluid persisted. Other studies show that bacteria can be found in the middle ear fluid of only 21 to 25 percent of children who do not respond to antibiotics.[66, 67] In this substantial number of children, it is likely that infection either never was or is no longer a consideration in their illness. The root of their problem may be increased susceptibility to infection or inflammation, due to an unknown cause.

The issue of whether bacteria cause otitis media or act as opportunists cannot be answered fully here. It is likely that under certain conditions, either may be true. There is no doubt that bacteria, viruses, and parasites exact a considerable toll on human health. Every effort should be made to reduce the suffering caused by these microbes. But if the individual child's susceptibility to infection is not considered, repeated infections and continued lowering of resistance may be the result in a significant number of children.

Mechanical Obstruction

Otitis media can occur when the eustachian tube is blocked, or obstructed, by physical or mechanical means. The most common factors associated with mechanical blockage of the eustachian tube are swollen tonsils or adenoids. It was this association that prompted the widespread use of tonsillectomy and adenoidectomy in the early days of treating ear infections. The cause of swollen tonsils or adenoids is not fully understood, but many doctors believe they can be caused or aggravated by allergies. Thus, allergies can lead to the development of one form of mechanical obstruction.

There is another form of mechanical obstruction that further contributes to the development of middle ear problems (and quite possibly the tonsilar and adenoid swelling in some children) called *bio*mechanical obstruction. Biomechanical obstruction refers to blockage that is due to problems involving the structural components surrounding the ear and eustachian tube. These include the bones of the cranium, the TMJ (or jaw joint), and the cervical spine (i.e., the bones of the upper neck).

In other words, abnormal function of the components of the jaw, the skull, and especially the neck can contribute to, and in some cases, cause the development of recurring ear problems.

Biomechanical problems often develop as a result of trauma at birth. Dr. F.R. Ford has pointed out that the spinal column of the infant is very different from that of an adult. He describes the infant vertebrae as a series of elastic cartilages surrounded by **inelastic** connective tissue.[68] This means that the tissue holding the infant's spine together does not lend itself to the same degree of flexibility or elasticity as adult tissue.

In addition, the infant has little or no muscle development. Muscular support of the head and neck is, therefore, non-existent. During birth, extremes of force are often used to pull, prod, or pry the newborn out of the birth canal. According to Dr. Abraham Towbin, of the Department of Neuropathology at Harvard Medical School, "During the final extraction of the fetus, mechanical stress imposed by obstetrical manipulation—even the application of standard orthodox procedures—may prove intolerable to the fetus." He further states that, "During active labor the spinal column, particularly the cervical portion, may be injured as the fetus is compressed and forced down the birth canal."[69]

Tractional forces as high as 67 pounds have been recorded during the delivery of babies. In a study of the tensile strength of the newborn spinal column, it was found that traction of 90 pounds was enough to cause separation and dislocation of the vertebrae, especially in the cervical region. Dr. J.M. Duncan, the principal investigator in this study, comments, "This [amount of tractional force] is probably far from being what most obstetricians would regard as a great force."[70]

These tremendous tractional forces applied during delivery often result in mild to moderate* soft-tissue injury to the components of the infant's spinal column, primarily in the region of the upper neck (which has the greatest range of motion). In many ways, this can be likened to a mild whiplash injury. This microtrauma can occur during prolonged or difficult labor, but is accentuated when forceps, vacuum extraction, or even C-section is used. What may be surprising is that similar trauma can occur even during "normal" delivery.

In 1966, Dr. Viola Frymann examined 1,250 newborns for evidence of mechanical problems resulting from birth. (These births were not even classified as traumatic.) Ten percent of the infants displayed evidence of severe visible trauma, and 78 percent had evidence of articular strains. Therefore, almost 90 percent of all infants demonstrated some degree of biomechanical stress from birth.[71]

The result of these types of injuries often includes swelling, muscle spasm, decreased circulation, restricted motion, and slight slippage, or movement, of the upper vertebrae relative to one another (called subluxation). These effects can go undetected for months or even years. The child may display

---

*Dr. Abraham Towbin has also found severe spinal cord and brainstem injury that occur as a result of obstetrical trauma even in so-called normal births. This is outside the discussion of this book.

no obvious signs of injury, yet may suffer from eye, nose, throat, and of course, *middle ear complaints*.

Birth trauma is not the only contributor to biomechanical problems. Children, as any parent has observed, are notoriously inquisitive. Their need for climbing and exploration is matched only by their unending energy. In the course of their explorations, bumps and bruises are sure to come. These occur because of falls off the couch, off the bed, down the stairs, or on the playground. The falls, while usually leaving no outward signs of injury, often result in mild strains of the upper spinal column. It is these minor strains that can lead to problems.

Consider the case of Mary. Mary began getting ear infections when she was nine months of age. When the first episode occurred, she was taken to the pediatrician for antibiotic therapy. The antibiotic appeared to have little effect and in about three weeks, the ear began to improve. The next ear infection occurred at 12 months. Again, antibiotics were used but there was no improvement in her condition until several weeks later.

At 15 months, another ear infection developed. On the recommendation of a close friend, the mother brought Mary to our clinic. It was evident from my examination that there were important functional changes in the upper neck that suggested an injury had occurred. More specifically, there was a lateral displacement of the first cervical vertebra. When I brought this to the mother's attention, she recalled that Mary had taken a nasty fall off the couch at about eight and a half months of age. The earaches began shortly thereafter.

I treated Mary using manipulation of the upper spine. She slept comfortably that night, by the next day was markedly improved, and within three days had fully recovered. She didn't develop another case of otitis media until she was two and one-half years old. When this occurred, the mother brought Mary into the office, I treated her once, and the earache resolved in a few days.

In this case, the mother had breastfed Mary for one full year. Solid foods were introduced at nine months, and Mary's diet would, by many parents, be considered enviable in terms of its purity and quality. Even so, the ear infections occurred. Mary's earaches were the result of a structural problem. This problem would be unlikely to respond to antibiotics, tubes, or any number of other approaches—including some of the alternatives I'll be discussing. A structural problem requires a structural solution.

Gottfried Gutmann, M.D., one of Europe's most prominent researchers in the field of physical medicine, describes a case of an 18-month-old boy with early relapsing tonsillitis, frequent enteritis, and therapy-resistant conjunctivitis. The child also suffered from frequent earaches, colds, rhinitis, and sleep problems. The boy's birth had been normal, but he had fallen off the changing table several times.

Examination revealed kyphosis (a reverse curvature) between the second and third cervical vertebrae, and forward and lateral displacement of the first cervical vertebra (C1). After the first specific adjustment of C1, the child improved markedly. Within a short time his ear, nose, and throat problems had ceased.

Dr. Gutmann has reported on the examination and adjustment of more than 1,000 infants and children. His results show that blocked nerve impulses, which result from distortions in the occiput (base of the skull) and the first and second cervical vertebrae, contribute to many clinical conditions, ranging from central motor impairment to lowered resistance to infection. He states that increased susceptibility to infection of the *ear, nose, and throat* is one of the most common consequences of these upper cervical problems.[72, 73, 74]

Patricia C. Brennan, Ph.D., has recently shown that the activity of two types of white blood cells (known as neutrophils and monocytes) can be enhanced using spinal manipulation. With enhanced function, these cells are more efficient at killing bacteria.[75] This lends support to Dr. Gutmann's contention that biomechanical problems adversely effect immune function and that correction of these problems may have a beneficial effect on immune function.

These are significant findings. If true, they would suggest that many children who receive antibiotics and tubes do so unnecessarily. Not only do they receive needless therapy with their associated risks, but an important potential contributor to ongoing health problems goes untreated.

How important are biomechanical problems to the health of children? Gutmann recommends that examination of the upper cervical spine be mandatory after every difficult birth. In this way, when problems are found, they can immediately be corrected by manipulation (also called adjustment). The child who is two, four, or five and suffering from recurrent ear infections also should be examined for biomechanical problems. In the words of Gutmann, in children with recurrent infections due to biomechanical problems ". . . the success of adjustment overshadows every other type of treatment, especially the pharmaceutical approach."[76]

Biomechanical problems contribute to the development of middle ear infection through a series of events that begin with the vertebral column. The three uppermost structures of the spinal column are the second cervical vertebra (C2), the first cervical vertebra (C1), and the occiput (the base of the skull). These vertebrae are not only in proximity to the eustachian tube and tonsils, but they lie directly adjacent to major nerve cell centers called ganglia.

It is through these ganglia that nerve fibers of the autonomic nervous system must pass to get to their destination. The autonomic nervous system controls the automatic functions that go on daily, most of which you are unaware, including things like secretion of mucus and the formation of tears.

When there is a mechanical problem with the upper cervical vertebrae, the pressure, inflammation, and swelling produced around these ganglia, or nerve cell clusters, causes them to fire abnormally.[77] Dr. Chung Ha Suh, at the University of

Colorado, has demonstrated that a tiny amount of pressure on a nerve fiber is enough to alter its function by as much as 60 percent.[78] Aberrant signals from the autonomic nervous system lead to disrupted function, such as increased mucus secretion and altered blood flow in the body parts that the nerves supply. This includes the nasal cavity, the throat, the ears, and many others.

Dr. J. Seifert, of West Germany, reports that nearly 80 percent of children are not in autonomic balance, meaning that there is some form of interference with the normal functioning of the autonomic nervous system. This interference is commonly due to subluxation of the upper cervical vertebrae. Seifert bases this contention on his studies of the upper cervical spine in newborns and infants.[79]

Not only do biomechanical problems affect the nervous and immune systems, but they can contribute to impaired drainage of the lymphatic vessels. The lymphatic system is a network of vessels designed to carry immune cells and metabolic waste products away to the liver to be reprocessed. When biomechanical problems interfere with this process, the tonsils and adenoids (really just large lymph nodes), which are already working overtime to fight a local infection, cannot effectively discharge their waste products. This not only limits their infection-fighting capability, but it encourages them to remain swollen, further adding to the congestion of the eustachian tube.

Biomechanical Problems May Contribute to Otitis Media by:

- Causing autonomic nervous system interference.
- Impairing the lymph drainage from the tonsils and adenoids.
- Inhibiting the local immune response.

As we begin to understand the links between the nervous system and the immune system, it is clear that an ongoing feedback exists. Cells of the immune system relay messages to the nervous system by way of the chemicals they secrete, while the nervous system relays messages to the immune system by way of neurotransmitters. Interruption of the flow of information results in changes in function.

To understand the importance of nerve supply, consider the importance of blood supply. When the blood supply to the heart is slowly reduced over time, the efficiency of the heart muscle begins to decline. If the blood supply is abruptly interrupted, as in a heart attack, the heart tissue supplied by the vessels that have been blocked will die. Nerve fibers supply information to the parts of the body with which they connect. When nerve conduction is interfered with, the structures that the nerves supply are damaged as a result.

When biomechanical problems affect the upper cervical spine, this interferes with the nerve fibers that emanate from those levels of the spine. This is not a simple bone on a nerve interference, but a complex response of the tissues surrounding the nerves to the insult of biomechanical forces. Because of this interference, the structures these nerves supply in the ear, nose, and throat suffer from impaired function. The impaired function may include deficiencies in local immune function and changes in blood flow, which encourage swelling, increases in mucus secretion, and delayed healing.*

No one is certain of the extent to which biomechanical problems cause or contribute to otitis media. The findings of Dr. Gutmann, Dr. Frymann, and others suggest that in children with otitis media who have suffered trauma at or after birth, the prospect of biomechanical stress should be seriously considered. In the otitis-prone child who does not respond to other therapies, biomechanical stress should be considered, whether there has been physical trauma or not.

---

*Controlled studies are currently underway that will assess the role of manipulation in the treatment of otitis media and the role of manipulation in stimulating immune function.

Nutritional Deficiency

Over the past two decades, our understanding of nutrition has expanded rapidly. For instance, we know that a child's intake of dietary fats can either enhance or impair immune function. Intake of the wrong types of fats not only predisposes a child to developing recurrent infections, but to inflammatory conditions as well. Deficiency of certain trace elements and vitamins causes a child's metabolic machinery to go awry, even if essential fats are taken in proper proportion. If all is well regarding the intake of vitamins, minerals, and fats, there are still a host of dietary factors that can upset the balance.

These are important considerations in childhood ear infections. Understanding them can allow you to avoid some things that put your child at risk to ear infections and to do those things that will optimize your child's resistance to disease in general. In this section, we'll explore:

- Types of dietary fats and their sources.
- How fats are made into important substances that affect inflammation and immune function.
- The adverse effects of non-essential fats.
- The role of vitamins and minerals.
- How these factors interact to cause ear infections.
- How aspirin and acetaminophen (found in Tylenol) can aggravate infection and inflammation.

The information in this section is perhaps the most important tool to developing a better understanding of the role of diet and nutrition not only in regard to ear infections but illness of other types as well. For this reason, I have provided a substantial amount of background information.

Essential Fatty Acids and Dietary Fat

As I discuss the role of dietary fats in middle ear infections, keep in mind that the infant fat requirement is roughly 50 percent of total calories. This is because all developing cells, including those of the nervous system, consist of different types of fats. As a child ages, the fat requirement gradually decreases, eventually reaching about 25 percent of total calories by adulthood. Therefore, the types of fats eaten are especially crucial to an infant or toddler. When a child does not consume fats in the proper ratios, it can spell trouble that will last throughout childhood and even into adulthood.

There are two main types of dietary fats—called **saturated*** fats and **unsaturated*** fats. Saturated fats are those that we typically associate with conditions like heart disease. These fats are solid at room temperature. This is why butter, which is primarily saturated fat, remains solid when left out on the counter top. Your child's body needs certain saturated fats, but can make what it needs. Some saturated fats are useful and some interfere with the body's use of unsaturated essential fats.

Unsaturated fats are liquid at room temperature and are the main constituents of vegetable oils. As with saturated fats, your child's body can make most of what it needs, except linoleic and alpha-linolenic acid. These two are known as essential fatty acids—or EFAs. They are essential because they're necessary for survival and must be obtained through the diet. (Our bodies cannot make them.) Essential fatty acids are found in foods such as safflower and flax seed oil.

---

*The reason for the designation saturated and unsaturated is that chemically a saturated fat contains only *single* bonds, rendering them more stable, less reactive, and solid at room temperature. Unsaturated fats contain *double* bonds, which make them alterable by heat, light, other molecules, and air. They are therefore less stable, more reactive, and liquid at room temperature.

Besides the two essential fatty acids, there are a variety of non-essential fatty acids in our food. Non-essential fatty acids include those that your child's body can make and those that are artificially created through food processing. Much of the fats found in pastries and doughnuts are non-essential fatty acids created in the deep-frying process.

These artificially created fatty acids can do great harm once inside the body. The problem is that non-essential fatty acids comprise a substantial percentage of most children's diets today.

The Helpful Fatty Acids

There are two main families of essential fatty acids. These are called omega-6 and omega-3 fatty acids.

Omega-6 Fatty Acids. Linoleic acid (LA) is one of the chief EFAs in the omega-6 family. It is found in sunflower, safflower, corn, sesame, flax, soybean, and pumpkin seed. Safflower oil is the highest in LA. **Gamma linolenic acid** (GLA) is found in oil of evening primrose, borage oil, and mother's milk. GLA can be made from LA. Under certain conditions (discussed later), the body cannot convert LA into GLA, in which case GLA must be obtained from the diet. **Arachidonic acid** (AA) is found in animal products such as meat, dairy, and eggs (the only vegetable source is a few select species of seaweed). Both arachidonic acid and gamma linolenic acid can be synthesized from linoleic acid.

Omega-3 Fatty Acids. The omega-3 family consists primarily of the essential fatty acid **alpha-linolenic acid** (LNA). It is found in pumpkin seed, flax, soybean, walnut, and in minor amounts in other plants. Flax is the most abundant source, containing 50 to 60 percent of its oil as LNA. LNA is a cold-weather oil found mainly in plants in temperate regions (because of its insulating ability).

Eicosapentaenoic acid (EPA) and **Docosahexaenoic acid** (DHA) are considered cold water marine oils and are found in mackerel, salmon, trout, tuna, cod, and sardines. Like LNA, EPA and DHA have insulating properties. EPA and DHA can be made by the body from LNA and are therefore non-essential. However, under conditions where important enzymes are impaired, LNA does not get converted. In these instances, EPA and DHA become essential and must be obtained from the diet. One reason cod liver oil has been so beneficial over the years is its high EPA and DHA content. Societies which live on diets high in EPA have lower rates of heart and inflammatory diseases.

Changes in Consumption Habits

Food processing practices over the past 100 years have caused the dietary ratio of omega-3 to omega-6 fatty acids to become seriously out of balance for most Americans. While omega-6 intake has remained largely unchanged, omega-3 intake has decreased by nearly 80 percent.[80]

The main reasons for this decrease in omega-3 fatty acid consumption are:

- Omega-3 fatty acids are lost through chemical hydrogenation. Hydrogenation is the process used to turn oil from a liquid to a solid. For example, to convert sunflower oil into sunflower margarine requires hydrogenation.

- 40 percent of omega-3 oils are lost from the increased consumption of southern oils, which are omega-6-rich and omega-3-poor. In the U.S., we consume large amounts of sunflower, safflower, and corn oil—high in omega-6 but low in omega-3.

- Destruction of omega-3 oils occurs when the germ is milled out of northern cereal grains.[81] Essential fatty acids are located primarily in the germ portion of the grains we eat. When grain is milled to make flour, the germ is separated and the endosperm—which is low in EFAs—is sold to consumers. This is one reason that refined (or white) flour products contribute to poor health.

- Fatty acids are easily destroyed by light, heat and air, contributing to an increase of rancid fats in the diet.

Why Your Child's Body Needs Essential Fatty Acids

Essential fatty acids are an important source of energy for your child's body. But when converted into a family of compounds known as **prostaglandins**, they are among the most potent and vital substances produced in the body. Prostaglandins are hormone-like chemicals that perform an array of functions, ranging from regulating blood clotting to creating inflammation. Many prostaglandins perform dual functions, such as enhancing immunity and regulating hormones. For every prostaglandin that performs one function, there appears to be another that performs the opposite function. This system of checks and balances is in place to ensure that the action of one family of prostaglandins does not get out of control. For example, one prostaglandin family promotes inflammation while another prevents inflammation. If inflammation were prevented entirely, healing would never occur. Yet if inflammation were allowed to proceed unchecked, serious tissue destruction would occur. Likewise, if immunity is stimulated without restraint, it can lead to a disease where the immune system attacks normal body tissue. If immunity is suppressed, we succumb easily to infection.

Prostaglandins are one reason that your child's intake of the proper dietary fatty acids is so important, because only certain types of fatty acids can be made into certain types of prostaglandins. What your child eats is exactly what his cells become. It determines whether he creates inflammation or pre-

Figure 8
Sources of Omega-6 and Omega-3 Fatty Acids*

Omega-6 Oils			Omega-3 Oils	
LA	*GLA*	*AA*	*LNA*	*EPA/DHA*
Corn Safflower Sunflower Sesame	Evening Primrose Mother's Milk Borage Pumpkin	Meat Eggs Cow's Milk Butter	Flax Walnut Soybean	Salmon Mackerel Herring Sardines Trout

vents it, fights disease or gets it.

Some important functions of prostaglandins are listed below:[87]

- Regulate fever.
- Affect tissue swelling.
- Affect allergies.
- Affect shrinking and swelling of nasal mucous membranes.
- Regulate secretions and their viscosity.
- Cause pain or stop it.
- Regulate smooth muscle (such as those in the ear and those that control the eustachian tube).

---

*Most oils contain a mixture of LA, LNA, and other fatty acids These listings are to show those with the highest content of the fatty acid indicated. Note also that animal products are the only source of AA. LA = linoleic acid; GLA = gamma linolenic acid; AA = arachidonic acid; LNA = alpha linolenic acid; EPA = eicosapentaenoic acid; DHA = docosahexaenoic acid.

How EFAs Are Made Into Prostaglandins

There are three main families of prostaglandins, called PG1, PG2, and PG3. Linoleic acid (LA) is converted into PG1, arachidonic acid (AA) into PG2, and alpha-linolenic acid (LNA) into PG3. PG1 tends to control inflammation and enhance immunity. PG2 comprises a family of chemicals that are highly inflammatory and immune-suppressing. PG3 compounds tend to be anti-inflammatory. It is useful to think of PG1 and PG3 as "good guys" and PG2 as "bad guys." (This designation is technically incorrect since all prostaglandins carry out important functions.)

PG1
- blocks allergic response
- prevents inflammation
- improves nerve function
- enhances immune function

PG2
- stimulates allergic response
- promotes inflammation
- suppresses immune function

PG3
- blocks release of PG2 inflammatory precursors
- enhances immune function
- prevents inflammation

Essential fatty acids are converted into prostaglandins through a series of steps that require enzymes and co-factors (see figure 9). The main enzyme is known as d-6-d (delta-6-desaturase). Among the co-factors are vitamins A, B6, C, folic acid, and the trace elements zinc, copper, and magnesium. When these factors are present along with the proper fatty acids, the enzymes work to convert fatty acids into prostaglandins. If the co-factors are not present in sufficient amounts, the enzyme doesn't work, and essential fatty acids are not converted into prostaglandins. Even when the co-factors are present, the

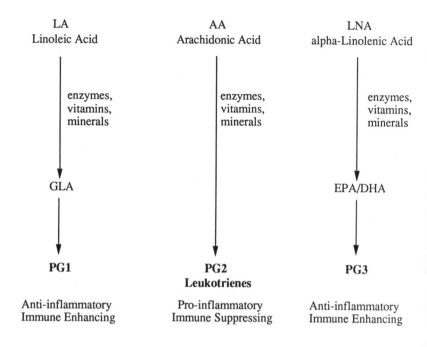

Figure 9

How Dietary Essential Fatty Acids are Converted Into Prostaglandins

*The description of prostaglandins as pro- or anti-inflammatory, or immune enhancing or suppressing is an oversimplification of what actually occurs. However, these designations are useful to show the general way in which these substances affect the body.

enzymes can be prevented from working normally by many factors that are abundant in our children's diets today.

Fatty Acids and Breastmilk

One reason breastfeeding is critical to infant and child health is the ratio of essential fatty acids it contains. One important fat found in breastmilk is GLA, or gamma linolenic acid. This is not an essential fatty acid for most adults. However, in infants the enzyme that converts dietary linoleic acid (LA) into GLA is inactive. Breastmilk supplies the needed GLA until the infant's metabolism begins to activate the enzyme on its own. Once this occurs, GLA from the diet is not as crucial.

GLA is necessary for the production of the anti-inflammatory PG1s. If the infant's diet does not contain sufficient amounts of GLA, sufficient PG1 will not be made. If PG1 is not produced in adequate amounts, there is little to oppose the immune-suppressing and inflammation-producing effects of PG2s. Breastmilk also contains the omega-3 fatty acid alpha-linolenic acid (LNA).

Mothers who breastfeed should be aware that the fatty acid content of their diet reflects directly what their breastmilk will contain. If the diet is deficient in omega-3 fatty acids, the breastmilk will be low as well. Worse, if a nursing mother's diet is high in saturated, partially hydrogenated, or trans fats (discussed later), the suckling infant will ingest them and be subjected to all the adverse consequences of exposure to these substances. These non-essential fats show up in mother's milk within 24 hours of the time they were eaten.

The breastmilk of American women tends to be far lower in essential fatty acids than is the breastmilk of women from non-industrialized nations such as Nigeria. Nigerian women consume unprocessed food, which is higher in needed fatty acids and co-factors.[83]

Breastmilk is also a nursing child's only source of zinc, which is essential to proper utilization of fatty acids. During pregnancy and lactation, a mother's zinc requirement increases. It is important that dietary levels of zinc be adequate while breastfeeding to ensure that the baby receives adequate amounts. Recent evidence shows the average nursing mother may only be getting 42 percent of the recommended daily allowance for zinc.[84]

How Non-Essential Fats Contribute to Illness

Non-essential fatty acids are present naturally in the food we eat. They are also created through food processing. It is those created through food processing that I focus on here. Fatty acids are very sensitive to heat, light, and oxygen. Exposure of oil to heat and air, such as in frying, results in the formation of substances called free radicals.

Free radicals are highly reactive chemical species that can be likened to a lighted match dropped on a dry forest floor. When the match is dropped, tiny twigs and leaves begin to burn. The fire grows and spreads in all directions. Burning embers leap from tree to tree, setting other areas of the forest ablaze in a chain reaction. Eventually large areas of forest are burned. The blaze continues to damage the forest until rainfall occurs or firefighters arrive to spray water on it.

Free radicals released through frying cause chain reactions in the oil molecules, altering their physical shape and chemical usefulness. The resulting chemicals include toxic byproducts about which we know very little. When these chemically altered fats are ingested, they alter the structure of cell membranes, and can trigger chain reactions such as that in the forest. One byproduct created through the cooking and hydrogenation of oil is called the **trans fatty acid**.

Trans fatty acids have a number of adverse effects on the body. They are solid at body temperature, whereas the "good" fatty acids (called cis*) are liquid. They are far more sticky than the "good" fatty acids so they can cause fatty deposits in the blood vessels, liver, and other organs. Normal essential fatty acids are "U" shaped, and are thus recognized by the body's enzymes and incorporated into the design of all body cells. Trans fatty acids are "arrow" shaped and cause serious irregularities in the cell structures. These arrow-shaped fats can

---

*The designation *cis* and *trans* refers to the side of the double bond on which the carbon chains reside. *Cis* literally means "on this side." When the chains are on the same side, the fat molecule is "U" shaped. *Trans* means "across." When the chains are across from one another, the fat molecule is "arrow" shaped. All naturally occurring unsaturated fatty acids are *cis*—this is the form the body must have.

slip into the body without being metabolized. They then stick to body tissues rather than being burned as energy.

Trans fatty acids change the permeability of cell membranes. Therefore, things that should get into the cell often don't, and those that shouldn't often do. This latter point is very important because the cell membrane is a vital barrier that protects cells from invading chemicals, bacteria, and viruses.

Trans fats also have a negative impact on the nervous system. Since the nervous system consists primarily of fat tissue, excess trans fatty acids can cause degeneration of nerves and change their electrical properties. This results in abnormal signals being sent from place to place. However, the most damaging effect of trans fatty acids is their ability to cause damage to the existing good fatty acids and drastically alter the production of prostaglandins. (This will be described later in the chapter.)

High levels of trans fats in the diet of children is especially worrisome because once incorporated into the tissues, trans fats are extremely difficult to remove. It takes more than seven weeks to remove half of the trans fats from the heart, and nine days to remove half from the liver.[85] If trans fats continue to be eaten, the residue continues to build and build over time. This gradually changes the composition of the body cells, making them rigid, sticky, and susceptible to damage (such as inflammation and infection). The only presently known way of removing trans fats from the body is to consume omega-3 fatty acids with the needed co-factors (meanwhile reducing the intake of trans fats).

Trans fatty acids comprise an alarming 10 percent of American's daily fat intake. The most common source is hydrogenated products like margarine and shortening that come from partially hydrogenated vegetable oils. Your child's diet is full of trans fatty acids. Several research studies conducted in the 1980s have shown the trans fatty acid content of common foods to be as high as 60 percent of the total fat with almost no essential fatty acids (the "good" fats) present. For instance,

Food Source	% of Fat as Trans Fatty Acids*
	Figure 10
	The Trans Fatty Acid Content of Common Foods
Breads and Rolls	1.8–24
Cakes and Cookies	30–40
Candy and Frostings	38.6
Crackers	20–30
French Fries	37.4
Margarine	
Hard	6–47.8
Soft	6–17
Pastries	33.5
Vegetable Shortening	37.3
Corn Chips	24–30

Journal of the American Oil Chemical Society, Vol. 60, 1983.[89]
Nutrition Reviews, 1984.[90]

*Less than 1 or 2 percent trans fatty acids is ideal.

up to 31 percent of the fats in stick margarine are trans fats. (Because of the dangers of trans fats, the Dutch government has banned the sale of margarines containing trans fatty acids.) Vegetable oil shortenings often contain over 37 percent trans fats. Vegetable salad oils contain up to 13.7 percent. French fries are as high as 37.4 percent. Candies, frostings, cakes, and cookies all contain anywhere from 30 to 40 percent of their fats as trans fats. Bakery products such as doughnuts, some breads, and rolls contain as high as 33.5 percent trans fatty acids.[86, 87]

According to research compiled in the book *Fats and Oils*, we consume about 40 grams of margarine and shortening per day (by direct consumption and indirect consumption such as in the products mentioned above).[88] The trans fatty acid content of these substances is dangerously high and is contributing to many chronic infectious and inflammatory illnesses experienced by Americans—including middle ear infection.

A trip to the local fast food joint can fill your child up with significant amounts of trans fatty acids.* Consider the typical meal ordered at one of these establishments: Cheeseburger, french fries, and a cola. The cheese, if real, contains saturated fats; if artificial, it contains partially hydrogenated fats. The hamburger, besides containing high amounts of saturated fats, is one of the richest sources of arachidonic acid (the one that if present in excess can lead to inflammation). The french fries (or anything deep-fried including potato cakes, fish sandwiches, chicken nuggets), as I showed earlier, may contain almost 40 percent of their fat as trans fatty acids. The cola is high in sugar and caffeine, and contains substances that deplete magnesium. (See chapter 7.) Not only is this meal almost 50 percent fat, but as much as 40 percent of the fat may be in the form of trans fatty acids. One of these meals is not likely to harm anyone. However, one, three or five times a week may contribute to chronic health problems.

How does this type of food affect inflammation and immune function? Think about what you've learned about fatty acids and prostaglandins. To begin with, the high amounts of trans fatty acids and the depletion of magnesium blocks the enzyme needed to produce the prostaglandins that are anti-inflammatory and immune-stimulating. In addition, high levels of arachidonic acid in the meat favor the formation of the inflammatory and immune-suppressing prostaglandins (since AA is the main precursor for these compounds). Trans fatty acids also trigger the release of arachidonic acid from cells, which initiates the release of inflammatory substances. Unless measures are taken to reduce this type of eating, we only con-

---

*Even foods labeled "all natural" or "contains no additives or preservatives" often contain hydrogenated oils and trans fats.

tinue to set the stage for illness. Unfortunately, almost every aspect of our children's diets contain altered fatty acids.

Protective Nutrients

Protecting us from the ravages of free radicals and non-essential fats is the **antioxidant defense system**. The anti-oxidant defense system consists of nutrients, including beta-carotene, vitamin C, and vitamin E. Two other powerful anti-oxidants, glutathione and superoxide dismutase, require selenium and riboflavin, and copper, zinc and manganese, respectively. The anti-oxidant defense system can be likened to the rainfall or firefighters described in the above analogy.

When our cells are exposed to free radicals, some local damage occurs. If the anti-oxidant defense system is operating at its peak, the free radicals are "quenched" and produce no more damage. The tissue is repaired and all proceeds well. This is a normal occurrence and goes on constantly within the body. However, if the free radical is not "quenched"—due to a deficiency of one or more of the anti-oxidant nutrients, or an excess of altered fatty acids—a chain reaction begins that can lead to damage throughout the cell. This damage often manifests as inflammation.

Free-radical substances can enter the body from outside sources, including smog, indoor air pollutants, food, water, and radiation. Free radicals are also produced within the body through the normal activity of white blood cells. Our cell membranes are very susceptible to damage by free radicals (and trans fatty acids).

Why Your Child's Important Enzymes May Not Work

I earlier described the enzyme (called delta-6-desaturase) that can easily be prevented from working by either a lack of proper co-factor nutrients or the presence of certain inhibitory compounds in the diet. The presence of these inhibitory compounds can cause both the 1 and 3 prostaglandins to be blocked, leading to the release of only the 2 prostaglandins, or those that are inflammation-producing and immune-suppressing.

The substances that block this enzyme include:[91]

- Saturated fat in excess (typically animal fat, but also includes saturated warm weather oils such as coconut and palm kernel oil).

- Trans fatty acids (described elsewhere in this chapter).

- Oxidizing chemicals (including indoor air pollutants, and constituents of cigarette smoke).

- Aspirin, acetaminophen, and other anti-inflammatory drugs.

- Alcohol (cough syrups and other medications). (See chapter 8 for a discussion of FAS.)

- Cortisone (found in many topical creams, nasal sprays, and bronchial inhalers).

- Ionizing radiation (such as X-rays).

- High cholesterol (not a great problem with most children although in some communities up to 50 percent of the children are found to have cholesterol that is considered too high).

- Fasting. (Children usually do not fast, but in cases where the caloric intake is too low, the enzyme may be affected.)

- Refined sugar and flour. (The average American consumes more than 120 pounds of sugar per year.)

- Environmental pollutants (such as lead and cadmium).

- Atopy (an inherited susceptibility to certain diseases such as allergic rhinitis, eczema, and asthma). (More than 70 percent of hyperactive children come from atopic families.)

There are also certain conditions under which the enzymes function poorly. These include:

- Infancy. (The enzyme is not yet active.)
- Diabetes. (In these children, the enzyme is only about 1 percent active.)
- Stress. (Includes children experiencing emotional stress because of problems in the family, at school, day care, or with friends. Under stress, your child's adrenal glands release a stress hormone known as epinephrine, which prevents the enzyme from properly working.)

To function properly, the enzyme requires the presence of certain nutrients in adequate amounts. Included are:

- Magnesium
- Zinc
- Vitamin B6
- Selenium
- Beta-carotene
- Insulin
- Protein
- Vitamin C
- Vitamin B3
- Vitamin A
- Copper

A Trend of Vitamin and Mineral Deficiencies

The diet of the average American child is commonly full of calories and lacking in nutrients. The responsibility for this unfortunate situation lies equally with parents, food manufacturers, advertisers, food growers, and even doctors (because of their general lack of training in nutrition).

Heavy dependence upon chemicals in the growth of food is a substantial contributor to the poor nutrient content of our food. The magnesium content of food is reduced even before processing, due to the use of potassium fertilizers in agriculture.[92] Nutrient levels of food can vary greatly from region to region. For instance, the beta-carotene content of carrots may vary many-fold depending upon the area of the country in which the carrots have been grown.

Processing of food adds substantially to lowered nutrient content. The trace element magnesium is often found in short supply in the diet of American children. Magnesium is critical for proper fatty acid metabolism, but high intake of *saturated* fat increases the body's excretion of magnesium in the urine.[93] Magnesium is located in the germ of most grains. When the grain is processed, the germ is usually discarded, and the endosperm is sold to consumers for use in flour, cereals, cake mixes, and a variety of food products. Processing removes roughly 85 percent of the magnesium from the grain.

Processing of grains also leads to the loss of vitamins B1, B2, B3, B6, E, and folic acid. Important trace minerals and essential fatty acids reside in the same portion of the grain as the vitamins. Thus, processing leads to the loss of selenium, zinc, linoleic acid, and alpha-linolenic acid as well. More than 20 nutrients are removed in the processing of flour. Of these, only 7 are replaced through fortification. Improper cooking methods often lead to substantial losses of folic acid, B-vitamins, and vitamin C.

According to Dr. Donald Rudin, anti-nutrients have increased significantly in the diet of Americans. Saturated fat has increased 100 percent, cholesterol 50 percent, refined sugar nearly 1,000 percent, salt nearly 500 percent, and "funny fat" isomers (including trans fatty acids) 1,000 percent.[94]

These changes in eating and food-processing practices have translated into deficiencies in the real world. In *The Selected Minerals in Food Survey* conducted by the FDA from 1982 to 1984, researchers found that daily levels of 11 essential minerals, including calcium, zinc, copper, and magnesium, were less than 80 percent of the RDA for some or all age groups. Among the groups at greatest risk of low intake were children.[95]

The Ear Infection Connection

There is direct evidence that deficiency of certain nutrients either increases the susceptibility to or causes otitis media. The reason for this is unclear, but it may be due in part to the need for these nutrients in fatty acid metabolism, which directly affects immune function and inflammation.

Vitamin A deficiency has been shown in animal studies to lead to otitis media. As I described earlier in this chapter, the middle ear is lined with column-shaped cells covered with tiny hairs called cilia. The cilia help to keep the allergens and bacteria from getting into the middle ear by trapping them and waving them down the eustachian tube to be eliminated. It appears that when vitamin A is deficient, the cells lining the middle ear and eustachian tube lose their cilia and become flattened out. When this occurs, the middle ear is not as effectively protected from infection. Vitamin A and beta-carotene (which is two molecules of vitamin A hooked together) are important co-factors in fatty acid conversion to prostaglandins.[96]

Zinc is another nutrient necessary for proper immune function and conversion of fatty acids. Children who are zinc-deficient suffer from atrophy (shrinkage) of the thymus gland.[97] The thymus gland lies directly behind the breastbone (sternum) and is the main source of T-lymphocytes, which are necessary for a child's cell-mediated immunity. Researchers in Sweden report that children who suffer from recurrent upper respiratory and ear infections are more likely to be zinc- (and iron-) deficient than their healthy counterparts.[98]

Several researchers have found that deficiency of various fatty acids in the cells (due to dietary deficiency) leads to abnormal production and release of immune-suppressing and inflammation-producing prostaglandins.[99] These prostaglandins have been shown to contribute to conditions such as rhinitis, asthma, eczema, and allergies.[100] Only recently have we come to realize that the same types of processes might contribute to the development of middle ear infection in children.

When the middle ear fluid of children with otitis media is analyzed, a wide range of inflammatory prostaglandins is typically found. Dr. David P. Skoner and his colleagues studied 102 patients who had persistent middle ear fluid that did not respond to antibiotic therapy. When the middle ear fluid was tested for several inflammatory compounds, Skoner found among them one of the 2-series prostaglandins in substantial amounts. Of these children with inflamed middle ears, only 21 percent had pathogenic bacteria in their middle ear fluid.[101]

At the Division of Otolaryngology-Head and Neck Surgery, at Loma Linda University, Dr. Timothy T.K. Jung conducted an extensive analysis of middle ear fluid for the presence of inflammatory compounds. His work indicates that high concentrations of some of the 2-series prostaglandins (PG2s) and leukotrienes (LTs) are present in the middle ear fluid of children with otitis media.[102]

Some medical researchers are using this information to find new drugs that might block the inflammatory process at various stages. While using anti-inflammatory drugs may be helpful in the short term, it does nothing to correct the underlying problems that set the stage for inflammation. Only by taking a careful look at diet and nutrition (since food provides the fuel for the inflammatory fire) can we hope to understand and correct the imbalances that contribute to otitis media in the immune and inflammatory systems.

This look begins with the fat arachidonic acid. Arachidonic acid is the omega-6 fatty acid found in meat, eggs, and milk. It also can be manufactured from linoleic acid, an omega-6 fatty acid derived from vegetable sources. Arachidonic acid is an important component of the membranes of all body cells. When arachidonic acid is released from the cells, it is quickly converted into a wide array of inflammatory substances—most notably prostaglandins (PGs) and leukotrienes (LTs). This is a normal part of the healing response, since these substances mobilize parts of the body defenses that repair tissue and fight infection. However, if this release of arachidonic acid—with its conversion to PGs and LTs—continues unchecked or is allowed to be triggered with minimal provocation, serious tissue injury can occur.

This is one reason that omega-6 and omega-3 fatty acids must be consumed in proper proportion. Excess arachidonic acid in the diet loads the cells with the fuel for inflammation. If omega-6 linoleic acid is present in excess relative to omega-3 fatty acids, some of the excess is converted into arachidonic acid and stored in the cell membranes. When omega-3 and omega-6 fatty acids are consumed in balanced amounts, 1) production of PG1s, which oppose PG2s, takes place adequately, 2) production of EPA occurs, which blocks the release of arachidonic acid, and 3) PG3 formation occurs, which blocks the action of PG2s and LTs.

Vitamins A and E also prevent the release of arachidonic acid from cells, acting as another buffer against excessive inflammation. Even if arachidonic acid is released, adequate levels of zinc and bioflavonoids can prevent it from being converted excessively into PG2s and LTs.

What are leukotrienes? Leukotrienes (LTs) are made from arachidonic acid. They are 1,000 to 10,000 times more inflammatory than histamine[103] (responsible for the runny nose, itchy eyes, and other symptoms associated with hay fever and allergy) and 1,000 times more inflammatory than the PG2 compounds.[104] Initially, leukotrienes are helpful because they signal the leukocytes (or white blood cells) to accumulate in an infected area.* However, excessive or prolonged secretion of these chemicals can spell disaster. Leukotrienes also produce asthma and hypersensitivity reactions.[105] They are potent inhibitors of immune cells called T-helpers, and potent stimulators of those called T-suppressors. They can, therefore, cause immune alteration when present even in minute quantities.[106] Leukotrienes stimulate secretion of mucus and are found in sig-

---

*Leukotrienes also perform a variety of other functions.

nificant amounts in children with otitis media (especially chronic or mucoid otitis media).[107]

The events that trigger the release of these compounds in the middle ear are often initiated by bacteria (when present), but can be triggered by free radicals, volatile pollutants, cigarette smoke (which contains both free radicals and volatile pollutants), viruses, trans fatty acids, or mechanical eustachian tube obstruction.*[108]

I described earlier how whatever your child eats (especially in terms of fats) is what his cells become. If the wrong types of fats have been consumed, the cell membranes will be made up of those fats. The cell membrane is the protective wall that surrounds every cell that lines the middle ear, eustachian tube, and the white blood cells that might be called upon to fight infection. When the events that trigger inflammation occur, arachidonic acid is released from the cells. If the proper balance of omega-3 and omega-6 fatty acids have been consumed (along with the supportive nutrients), inflammation usually proceeds only to the point necessary. However, if omega-6 fatty acids are consumed in excess or omega-3 fatty acids consumed in deficiency, the conditions are ripe for continued inflammation and tissue injury.

This may be why so many children continue to have inflammatory middle ear fluid in spite of round after round of antibiotics. In a substantial number of the children who do not respond to antibiotics, the middle ear fluid contains no bacteria.[109] The fluid is, however, filled with inflammatory substances. This suggests either that infection was never present, or that any infection might have long ago been eradicated, leaving the underlying inflammatory changes in its wake. What is likely

---

*It is interesting to note that mechanical eustachian tube obstruction can trigger the release of inflammatory compounds in the middle ear. This may be one reason that spinal manipulation has been useful in managing otitis media in some children (since manipulation can contribute to the reversal of mechanical obstruction).

needed in these children is dietary and nutritional intervention to correct the deteriorating imbalance in the inflammatory system.

Why Aspirin and Acetaminophen Can Cause Problems

Aspirin and acetaminophen have long been used to control fever, relieve pain, and reduce inflammation associated with otitis media. For many years, the reasons for the action of these drugs were not well understood. Today we know that aspirin (and acetaminophen—Tylenol) are *prostaglandin inhibitors*, meaning that they reduce inflammation by blocking the formation of inflammatory prostaglandins. Unfortunately, there is a substantial trade-off. Aspirin interferes with the enzymes that convert arachidonic acid (AA) into PG2, which on the surface is helpful since PG2 is inflammation-producing. However, aspirin also interferes with the enzymes that convert LA into the anti-inflammatory PG1 and LNA into the anti-inflammatory PG3—this is not good. In other words, anti-inflammatory drugs block the formation of *some* chemicals that promote inflammation, but they also block those that naturally prevent inflammation.

A principal drawback of these drugs is that by blocking the formation of one family of inflammatory substances, the formation of another family of compounds is favored. Members of this family, known as leukotrienes,* are generally more inflammatory than those that aspirin or acetaminophen are used to block. Thus, aspirin or acetaminophen can favor the release of substances that make inflammation worse. (See chapter 8 for more information and diagrams.)

---

*Note: Inflammatory HPETEs and related compounds are often produced along with leukotrienes. HPETEs are also found in substantial amounts in inflamed or infected middle ear fluid. They have been left out of the above discussion for reasons of simplicity.

This has recently been confirmed by the research of Dr. Timothy T.K. Jung, who showed that when drugs such as aspirin and acetaminophen are used to treat middle ear infection, the inflammation actually gets worse. Dr. Jung states, "It is conceivable that the free use of aspirin for children with acute otitis media may contribute to the development of mucoid otitis media in these children."[110] Mucoid otitis media is a chronic and therapy-resistant form of middle ear disease where the fluid is very thick and sticky.

The adverse effect of anti-inflammatory drugs on the production of highly inflammatory leukotrienes also would explain, in part, the study shared earlier which showed that children with chicken pox recover more slowly when acetaminophen is used.

Cortisone is another drug used by some doctors in the treatment of otitis media (sometimes as nasal spray). Cortisone blocks inflammation by preventing the release of arachidonic acid, thereby preventing both PG2s and LTs from being formed. However, it also blocks the enzymes needed in the formation of the "good" prostaglandins. In addition, cortisone promotes depletion of zinc.[111] Thus, the long-term effect of using cortisone tends toward the suppression of the body's natural inflammation-fighting machinery.

Based on the available research, it appears that a substantial portion of children suffering from recurrent infections and inflammation may do so because of improper intake of essential fatty acids (and some additional nutrients). Given the ability of aspirin and other anti-inflammatory drugs to *increase* inflammation by further aggravating fatty acid problems, it seems more prudent to restrict the use of these drugs and focus our efforts on correcting the cause of the inflammation.

* * *

As the role of nutrition in both inflammation and immune function becomes more clear, the prospects for therapy based on nutritional and dietary intervention improve. It is likely that many children now using antibiotics and tubes might avoid them with proper nutritional care. Even under circumstances in which antibiotics or tubes are used, careful nutritional management will enhance recovery and may reduce the need for further intervention. The key to this is to demand that your doctor understand the intricacies of nutritional therapy. Children with otitis media should to have a thorough assessment of their dietary intake and nutritional status performed.

Solutions to the nutritional problems presented in this section will be discussed in chapters 6, 7, and 8.

In Summary

The evidence presented in this chapter lends strong support to the contention that childhood otitis media is a complex and multifactoral problem. It is rare that all the factors discussed in this chapter are present in a given child. What is not uncommon, however, is to find a dynamic interplay bewteen two or more of these factors. For example, deficiency of fatty acids can predispose a child to allergies. Allergies predispose some children to otitis media. Once the allergic syndrome is set in motion, both nutritional intervention and allergy management must be employed to treat the earaches effectively.

Understanding the causes of otitis media is essential to developing effective treatment. If middle ear fluid is due to factors described above, antibiotics and surgery can only be considered palliative (or symptom-reducing) measures. There will be instances when antibiotics and surgery are required, but it would be prudent for all doctors to recognize the need to address those factors that lead to the development of middle ear fluid and infection.

Chapter 6

Home Care for Earaches

"Parents have reported to me that after learning self-care, they are able to cut their visits to the doctor by up to 85 percent." [1]

George Wootan, M.D.

Taking responsibility for home care or choosing to use alternative forms of health care is not a substitute for conventional medical care. As Dr. Richard Moskowitz says, it calls for "a different relationship to the healing process and the health-care system, based on personal choice and direct participation. We still need help when our children get sick, and we need to know that this help is available to us." [2]

It's important that you develop a relationship with a doctor who is at least somewhat supportive of your desire to use alternatives and home care methods. (Most doctors would agree that home care methods are useful if they are not taken to extremes and do not replace common sense.) Also of importance is a family environment where both you and your spouse share a common philosophical belief about how to care for your child. Without this, your desire to use alternatives or home care methods will often be met with confrontation. Therefore, it is important that you discuss ideas and share information.

When to Call the Doctor

Many childhood illnesses can be taken care of at home. But you should always be aware of the general signs that would indicate the need for a doctor. You are often the best judge of your child's condition. The most telling sign of serious illness is your child's behavior. If she looks ill, is behaving unusually, and your instincts tell you to take her in, then follow your instincts. The following guidelines are useful in helping to decide when to take your child to the doctor.

Get Medical Care Immediately:[3]

- If your child shows signs of extreme weakness or loss of consciousness.

- If there is a significant and abrupt change in your child's voice.

- If your child displays or complains of neck stiffness or headache.

- If your child has difficulty breathing or is vomiting.

Get Medical Care Today:

- Anytime a baby has discharge from the ear.

- If an acute earache does not respond to home care within 48 hours.

- If your child experiences a sudden loss of hearing.

- If your child experiences severe ear pain.

- If you see redness on or your child complains of pain around the bony structure behind the ear (known as the mastoid process).

- If fever fails to subside after three days.

- If your infant or toddler continually pokes her finger into the ear canal or tugs at the ear.

See Your Practitioner Soon:

- If a chronic earache has not responded to home care within two weeks.

- If ear discharge has persisted beyond one week.

- If hearing loss has persisted for more than one to two weeks.

Fever: Your Child's Friend, not Foe

Parents in this country tend to be overconcerned about fever in their children. In a 1980 survey, more than half of parents erroneously believed that a fever of 104 degrees or less could cause permanent brain damage. Roughly 85 percent gave fever-reducing drugs before temperatures reached 102 degrees, and 68 percent gave their children sponge baths before fever reached 103 degrees.[4, 5]

Contrary to these beliefs, elevated body temperature is an important sign that indicates the immune system is mounting an attack against an infectious agent. When fever is allowed to develop, the body is more efficient at fighting infection. When fever is suppressed, the recovery from illness is slowed.[6] For instance, infected animal pups that are prevented from raising their body temperature have a significantly higher rate of mortality than those that are allowed to raise their body temperature.[7]

Fever is increasingly being viewed as a controlled response to infection, by which the body raises the "set point" of its thermostat for a specific purpose. According to Matthew J. Kluger, Ph.D., of the Department of Physiology at the University of Michigan Medical School, elevated body temperature results in a modification of the levels of zinc and iron in the bloodstream, which significantly reduces the growth rate of pathogenic bacteria. In addition, fever enhances the bactericidal activity of white blood cells and increase their mobility.[8, 9]

A fever is generally considered high only after it rises to 105 degrees. In fact, the body will not allow a fever to rise above 106 degrees unless there is some rare factor present (such as in poisoning or encephalitis) that completely disrupts the body's thermal control mechanism. Fevers of 104 degrees and below are of little concern unless they persist for three or more days. Children commonly experience fluctuations in their *normal* daily temperatures of almost 2 degrees. The day begins with body temperature at its lowest. By late afternoon or evening, daily temperature has peaked.

This normal rise often gives parents the mistaken belief that a fever is rising. Even when fever rises, it gives no indication of the severity or progression of an illness.

There is a commonly held belief that if a fever rises too high, it can lead to febrile convulsions, and that febrile convulsions predispose a child to developing subsequent seizure disorders. However, convulsions occur in only a small percentage of children with high fever. In one study of 1,706 children who experienced febrile convulsions, there was no evidence of any motor defect and not one single death.[10, 11] There appears to be no evidence that febrile convulsions lead to the development of epilepsy.[12]

Fever-reducing drugs can complicate the healing process with sometimes serious consequences. Aspirin use can lead to the development of Reye's Syndrome, a fatal inflammation of the brain. Since this discovery, doctors no longer recommend aspirin for control of childhood fever. Instead, they recommend acetaminophen. I discussed the potential problems with using acetaminophen in chapter 5. According to Dr. Timothy Doran, ". . . we should be advising parents to treat the child and not the thermometer. If there's fever, and they [the child] are not uncomfortable with it, there is no reason to give it [acetaminophen]."[13]

Temperature can be taken by one of three methods: oral, axillary, or rectal. Taking the oral temperature of a young child is ill-advised because of the obvious risk of breaking the thermometer in the mouth. According to the late Robert S. Mendelsohn, M.D., the threat of rectal perforation (which is fatal in 50 percent of cases) while taking a rectal temperature is not worth the risk, so he advises taking an axillary temperature reading in children. Axillary temperature is usually about one degree lower than rectal temperature in an older child. In babies, the difference is negligible.[14]

According to Dr. Mendelsohn, fevers usually don't require medical attention, except:[15]

- If your child is less than two months old and his temperature exceeds 100 degrees.

- If fever fails to abate after three days or is accompanied by vomiting, respiratory distress, or persistent cough.

- If your child displays listlessness, irritability, or looks seriously ill.

- If your child is making strange twitching movements.

Keep Your Child At Home

There is nothing so disruptive to the healing process as being shuttled out of a comfortable and familiar environment. When a child is ill, she needs peace, quiet, the comforting words of a parent, a gentle touch, and most of all, the knowledge that during this time of discomfort and anxiety, her needs will be fully met. The purely physical needs of child such as providing food, water, medicine, and a change of bedding can be met by almost anyone. Typically a family member (usually a parent or grandparent) is needed to provide the intangibles that are such a large part of the healing response.

For a sick child, create an environment that is free of excessive stimulation. Keep the television and radio off. Dim the lights in the child's room or partially close the shade if the room is too bright. The room should be kept orderly. All toys should be in their place. Tell your child a comforting story. If you need to run errands, don't take your child with you. Wait until your spouse or a friend is available to help. Most of all, show your child extra love and attention, and think about how

comforting it was when you, as a child, were cared for by your
mother or father.

Avoid sending your sick child to school or day care.* These are environments that are highly stimulating and stressful to a sick child (not to mention the threat of spreading the illness to other children or "picking up something" from another child). A recent "solution" for working parents with sick children is the "day care infirmary"—a day care center staffed by medical personnel (usually nurses). While I can empathize with parents who cannot get off work to care for their sick child, I'm concerned about leaving a large number of moderately ill children together in such a setting.

When Your Child Must Be on Antibiotics

There may be instances when antibiotics will be necessary for your child. Under these circumstances, you must make every effort to minimize the adverse impact of the antibiotic on your child. The first step is to give a bifidus supplement (see section below on intestinal bacteria), one teaspoon, three times per day during the ten-day course of the antibiotic. Doses of bifidus should be given between doses of the antibiotic. In cases of sulfa drug therapy, a two- to three-hour spacing between the bifidus and antibiotic is recommended.[16] Once the antibiotic has been discontinued, continue to give bifidus for one full month.

You also should discuss with your doctor the prospects of your child taking Nystatin with the antibiotic. Nystatin is an antifungal agent that will prevent the overgrowth of intestinal yeast that often accompanies antibiotic therapy. Tell your doctor that you are aware that antibiotics can kill the beneficial bacteria which live in the intestine, and that when this occurs, there is nothing to keep the yeast organisms in check. Convey

---

*See chapter 7 for day care exclusion guidelines.

to him that you realize the need for antibiotics in this situation, but would like to take this additional step for your child. (Incidentally, years ago some antimicrobial preparations contained both antibacterial agents and Nystatin in the same tablet for the reason just mentioned.)

I also recommend that you neither accept nor request an antibiotic prescription over the phone. If your child is sick enough to require an antibiotic, he is sick enough to be seen by a doctor. A doctor cannot discern the state of your child's illness from a telephone call.

What If Your Doctor Recommends Adenoidectomy or Tubes?

Do not accept or reject surgery as a matter of course. If your child has had only a few ear infections and there are no signs of complications, you will want to approach the prospect of surgery with caution. Since ear infections are somewhat seasonal, I would be hesitant to agree to surgery if summer is just around the corner. If your doctor recommends tubes, remember that the likelihood of otorrhea (see chapter 3) is high during summer because of external contamination from swimming.

If your child has had recurrent earaches for some time that have not responded to any therapy, or there are signs of complications, you should consider tubes more realistically. In either case, I recommend that you get a second opinion from a doctor who is in no way associated with your doctor. Ask your friends and family to give you a recommendation, but don't get a referral from your doctor or his staff.

The ultimate decision rests with you. After you have considered all the evidence available to you and consulted with your doctors, you will need to decide what's best for your child. The information I presented in chapter 3 is not an indictment of tubes (or adenoidectomy) and I make no statement about the needs of an individual child. My intent is to present some hazards and complicating features of these procedures so that parents can weigh them against the potential benefits that might be afforded.

Climate Considerations

Fall, winter, and spring are seasons when ear infections are most common—winter being the most likely. An important consideration during these seasons is the relative humidity. In temperate regions such as Minnesota, the outdoor humidity in December falls to around 10 percent and below, while the indoor humidity can plummet to 0 to 5 percent. When the air is this dry, mucous membranes dry out rapidly, causing irritation of the upper respiratory tract, ear, nose, and throat. It will be important to take steps to humidify the air in your child's room. (Adequate fatty acid intake is also needed to maintain lubrication of the cell membranes.)

In contrast, regions such as San Francisco or Seattle become very damp and moist during mid-winter. Dampness also may contribute to upper respiratory and ear problems, but in a different way. If you live in an area like this, it will be important to maintain an area that is dry, warm, and free of excessive humidity. It also will be necessary to protect your child from the elements when going outside.

Emotional Factors

The emotional and physical bodies are not separate entities, but delicately interwoven. Physical distress can manifest emotional changes and emotional distress can manifest physical changes. Whenever illness strikes your child, be aware of emotional and developmental occurrences taking place in his life.

Observe whether your child is having struggles with peers. Is he frustrated trying to master a certain task? Is there a new sibling in the family competing for time and attention? Look at your interaction with your child. In the haste of your schedule, have you tended to rush him? Is your child's environment too restricted? Does your discipline reflect your needs or his? Have you recently divorced or separated? Do you have frequent arguments with your spouse? Have you or your spouse suffered from chronic illness that might be emotionally draining for your child? The list is endless. It is important that you are aware of the way in which events affecting the emotional well-being of your child affect his physical well-being.

I recall a training film designed to show the importance of doctors really getting to know their patients. (This film was based on a study of doctor/patient interaction compared with counselor/patient interaction.) In one segment, a father appears at the doctor's office with his young daughter who had been suffering from recurrent ear infections for six months. The pediatrician walked into the room, asked where the pain was, and proceeded to do an otoscopic exam of the ears. After viewing each ear for about thirty seconds, the doctor concluded that the girl was suffering from otitis media. He promptly prescribed an antibiotic and a decongestant, then left the room.

The study was designed so that a counselor would enter after the doctor had left. In this case, the counselor entered the room and began to ask about their family life. The father broke into tears within moments of beginning to tell how his wife had just died after a prolonged battle with cancer. It had taken a substantial toll on all the family members, especially the daughter. She developed her recurrent health problems while her mother was ill. The sad events of this story illustrate the importance of looking closely at events in our children's lives and listening carefully to not only the overt, but the more subtle signals as well.

A specific example of the relationship of emotion to disease deals with free will. As a child grows and develops emotionally, his will becomes more defined. The will to be an individual, the will to assert his strengths, the will to be free, the will to test limits, and so on, are the birthright of every child. While very powerful, the will of a child is extremely delicate and must be guided and nurtured. According to the principles of Chinese medicine, the will is housed in the kidneys. If the free will of a child is suppressed by a parent who asserts too much control, disciplines without consistency, or has unreasonable expectations, the will can be weakened. This, say the Chinese, results in diminished kidney energy. Because the kidneys influence the ears, diminished kidney energy easily manifests as ear problems. In many cases, it does not cause ear problems, but contributes greatly to increased susceptibility to them. According to Dr. Martha Benedict, a teacher and practitioner of Chinese medicine, roughly 25 percent of childhood ear problems have an emotional origin.

When my son was one year old, my wife and I decided it was time to move his crib into his own bedroom. I suspected this might be a traumatic event and was on the lookout for any unusual behaviors or symptoms. Caleb, who is rarely ill, awoke the next morning with a fever of 104 degrees. There were no other symptoms. During the next two days, we were careful to respond to all his needs and reassure him of our love and devotion. Within two days, things were back to normal with no need for any therapeutic intervention.

The key is to listen to your child and look at his life during times of illness. Meeting his emotional needs can be as important as meeting his physical needs!

Children with Down Syndrome

I noted earlier that roughly 60 percent of children with Down syndrome experience otitis media. This is one of the highest risk groups. The structure of the palate and nasopharynx creates an environment that is highly conducive to the development of congestion within the eustachian tube.

I have had minimal personal experience with Down syndrome children and cannot comment on the value of the home care methods or alternative treatment methods described in this book. However, recent evidence suggests that the defects in cellular immunity of children with Down syndrome can be corrected by oral zinc supplementation.[17, 18] This also may suggest that other nutrients would be of value in enhancing the immune response of these children. If you have a child with Down syndrome, I recommend you find a doctor who is knowledgeable in nutrition, and have a comprehensive evaluation of your child's nutritional status done.

In addition, there is evidence in the homeopathic literature that otitis media in Down syndrome can be managed well using the constitutional prescription of one of two homeopathic medicines. A description of these remedies is presented in chapter 8. (See *Baryta carbonica* and *Calcarea carbonica*.)

Signs of Diminished Hearing

Changes in hearing acuity may often be the only real signal that your child is having middle ear problems. Transient decreases in hearing are common with otitis media and are not usually cause for alarm. Chronic deficiencies in hearing are, of course, cause for concern and require attention.

Children who experience hearing loss are unlikely to alert you to it since they are frequently unaware of it themselves. When hearing changes occur, they are sometimes highly variable, fluctuating in severity from day to day.

Hearing changes in infants might be noticed by failure to respond to a loud noise or failure to turn their head to the side of a spoken voice. Older children may not respond to inquiries or respond frequently with "what?" or "huh?" They may have the volume on the television or radio turned up inordinately loud. A child who speaks more loudly than is normal also may suffer hearing deficiency.

Poor performance in school is sometimes a signal of hearing deficiency. There are instances where learning difficulties have been the only signal alerting parents or teachers to a hearing problem. Delayed speech and language is sometimes, but not always, an indicator of diminished hearing. If you feel there is a delay in your child's speech and language development, be sure to consult your doctor.

Remember, wax build-up in the ear canal can have a considerable muffling effect on incoming sound. When excessive wax is present in the ear canal, never attempt to remove it by inserting a cotton-tipped swab (or anything else for that matter). The risk of a perforated eardrum is not worth it. Instead, place a couple of drops of hydrogen peroxide (3 percent* as sold in drug stores) in the ear two to three times a day. This will gradually break up the mass of ear wax. Incidentally, excessive production of ear wax has been linked by some to deficiency of vitamin B6 or essential fatty acids. Thus, excessive ear wax may be an indicator of nutritional problems.

Foreign Bodies

Children are fond of placing tiny objects in their body orifices. The ear and nose are especially attractive. A foreign object placed in the ear canal can result in considerable pain if left long enough. Anything from peas to small buttons is fair game. Insects also can find their way into the ear canal. If you have reason to believe your child has put something in his ear, take him to the doctor for an examination.

Over the years, I've seen children who have stuffed all sorts of different objects up their nose. Peas and peanuts are favorites, but anything is possible. A foreign object in the nose can be the cause of persistent nasal discharge or offensive breath. I once examined a child who had a green, offensive nasal discharge of more than six months' duration. Previous doctors (who had apparently not examined the nasal cavity) had prescribed decongestants with no success. When the tiny piece of

---

*Some people have advocated taking hydrogen peroxide orally for a wide range of physical complaints. (I have no comment on this practice.) The mixtures used in such cases are usually 36 percent hydrogen peroxide. A mixture of this strength should NEVER be placed into the ear canal or on skin. The burns that result can be severe.

rubber band was finally removed, the boy's nasal discharge cleared up.

Home Care Methods

There are a variety of alternative treatment methods being used successfully to care for otitis media. In all cases, the methods of diagnosis and treatment are complex, requiring the expertise of a trained health practitioner. Home care methods based on the theme of these alternatives can be used with considerable success. Bear in mind that each child is different and not all will respond similarly to home care. One child may experience complete elimination of ear problems using home care methods, while another may notice little improvement.

It is advisable to consult your doctor before making changes in your child's diet or attempting any of the home care methods described below. The alternative methods of treating earaches include:

- Allergy Management.
- Acupuncture.
- Homeopathic Medicine.
- Botanical Medicine.
- Spinal Manipulation.
- Nutrition.

It may at first seem confusing to be presented with so many different approaches. The obvious question is, which approach should I use?

I don't advocate that you use all the home remedies with your child at once. The purpose of showing you this variety of approaches is to give you the opportunity to: 1) choose one that is comfortable to you and suits your personal philosophy, and 2) provide you with options should your child fail to respond to the first home care method you use.

Every child has specific individual needs. The key to helping your child is to individualize the care so it is precisely suited to him. Regardless of which home care methods you choose, you will want to make the necessary dietary changes and follow the prevention strategies that apply to your child's situation.

A rule of thumb is acute earaches respond more quickly, and chronic earaches respond more slowly. If your child has had recurrent infections, multiple courses of antibiotics, or tubes, recovery may be slower. In cases where tubes are used, you will find that healthy children often reject tubes soon after placement. Children who have a weaker constitution will often retain tympanostomy tubes for some time. If your child is among those who has retained the tubes for a long time, it will be important to build up his constitution. This takes time and often involves the help of a professional, although following the guidelines in this book will help immensely.

Allergy Management

Allergists have been around for decades so the treatment of allergy is nothing new. I discuss it as an alternative because conventional allergy management, which consists primarily of scratch testing and allergy shots, has been inadequate in meeting the needs of a large percentage of allergy sufferers. Allergists have also been surprisingly reluctant to acknowledge the existence of food allergy. According to Albert Rowe, M.D., "It is generally agreed that clinical allergy may exist in the absence of positive skin reactions, especially those to the scratch test. This is true primarily in food allergy and to a lesser extent in inhalant allergy."[19]

Shortly after I became aware of the role of food in ear infections, I treated a seven-year-old girl named Melody who suffered from severe exercise-induced asthma, recurrent tonsillitis, recurrent bronchopneumonia, and earaches. Because of the asthma, she was unable to walk a flight of stairs without becoming seriously short of breath and slept sitting up for many months. From age three and a half to age seven, Melody had been under the care of an allergist who routinely prescribed decongestants and antibiotics. The medication helped keep her out of serious distress, but there was little improvement in her condition.

My evaluation suggested that Melody was sensitive to dairy products and wheat. I recommended that her parents withhold these foods for six weeks. With some reluctance Melody's parents agreed to put her on the elimination diet. After one week, she began to improve. After six weeks, her ears were normal and her asthma improved. Remarkably, she was running and playing with no ill effects. Within two months, Melody was fully recovered, based on not only my evaluation, but that of her allergist as well.

What's interesting about this case is that Melody had gone through a full battery of allergy scratch tests that showed she was allergic to maple trees, dogs, cats, and horses—but no foods. Yet, as it turned out, Melody's recovery was based almost entirely on the removal of offending foods from her diet. The point is that no form of allergy testing is 100 percent accurate. Scratch testing frequently fails to identify allergies that exist. Blood testing is useful, but it also fails to identify some allergic children. Elimination-provocation testing (discussed below) is highly valuable, but has drawbacks as well. Because of this, some doctors are beginning to use a combination of tests to verify the presence of allergy. (See chapter 8 for types of allergy testing.)

If your child suffers from recurrent otitis media, you should consider allergy (or hypersensitivity) as a factor. Bear in mind that allergy is not a cause of disease, but the expression of some underlying weakness. Once the weakness is found and corrected, allergies frequently improve.

Ask the following questions to determine if allergy or sensitivity might be involved:

- Did the problems begin in the first six months of life?
- Did the problems start shortly after beginning solid foods?
- Did the problems start shortly after beginning formula?

- Do you or your spouse suffer from allergy or sensitivity?

- Does your child crave certain foods?

- Does the problem subside when traveling away from home?

- Does your child have irregular stools, colic, gas, diarrhea, or constipation?

- Does your child suffer from chronic rhinitis, or stuffy nose?

- Does your child have asthma, recurrent bronchitis, or other upper respiratory problems?

- Does the teacher notice changes in the child's behavior following lunch?

- Does your child develop symptoms following antibiotic therapy?

- Does your child have puffiness, dark circles, or "bags" under the eyes?

- Does your child have occasional difficulty hearing?

- Does your child have difficulty sleeping through the night?

- Does your child wet the bed (nocturnal eneuresis) either regularly or on occasion?

- Has your child been on allergy shots at any time in his/her life?

- Does your child suffer from eczema, dry scaly skin, or any other skin condition?

- Is your child overweight or underweight?

- Is your child a "fussy eater?" (Children with food allergies often lose their appetite or taste acuity.)

- Does your child have a horizontal crease on his/her nose or do the so-called "allergic salute?"

If the answer is "yes" to one or more of these questions, there is a chance that your child suffers from allergy or sensitivity to some substance and should be evaluated by a doctor.

Sometimes sensitivity to foods can be determined at home by performing an elimination-provocation test. The object of this test is to remove suspected offending foods from the diet for a period of time (elimination), observe for improvement, and then add the food back to see if the earache or other symptoms return (provocation).

If you are breastfeeding, it's important to examine your diet. First remove any drugs or vitamins from your diet and observe for improvement in your baby. Then remove the common offending foods (listed below) and observe for improvement. After five to seven days, if there is no improvement in your child's condition, your diet is probably not at fault. The problem is likely 1) related to your baby's diet (if on solids or some formula), 2) related to an airborne allergy, or 3) unrelated to allergy.

To test an older child, place her on a diet that is free of the common offenders. This includes:

- Dairy products, including milk, butter, cheese, yogurt, cottage cheese, cow's milk formula, and ice cream.

- Wheat, including not only bread and cereal, but anything that contains wheat such as gravies, crackers and cookies.

- Eggs or anything containing eggs.

- Chocolate.

- Citrus, especially oranges and orange juice.

- Corn, or anything containing corn, such as corn flakes.

- Soy. This is especially a problem with infant formula. Dr. William Crook states that 25 percent of infants with milk allergy develop allergy to soy.

- Peanuts, and other nuts. Peanut butter is a great favor-

ite among children and a frequent contributor to childhood health problems.

- Shellfish.
- Sugar.
- Yeast.

In place of these foods, feed your child lamb, rice,
squash, carrots, red potatoes, chicken, and applesauce. Observe
for improvement in ear symptoms, behavior, runny nose, cough,
or any other chronic symptom your child may display. After
five days, begin reintroducing the foods one at a time, beginning with those at the top of the list. Dairy products must be
avoided for at least three weeks before a determination about
sensitivity can be made. Only feed one food per meal, and give
the same food for three meals that day. Feeding more than one
will confuse the results. When you introduce a food, look for
a return of symptoms. Once a child has been off a food for
several days, the reaction upon reintroducing can be dramatic.

After you have tested all the foods, you will have an indication of the foods to which your child is sensitive. These
foods should be omitted from the diet for several months or
until long after the earaches have improved. Remember, earaches are a complex problem. Removing offending foods may
lead to striking improvement in some children and no improvement in others. (Note: Children with airborne allergies will
often experience a dramatic improvement in their airborne
allergies once their food allergies have been addressed.)

A special note should be made about yeast. Many children with recurrent earaches have been on prolonged or multiple courses of antibiotics in their lifetime. Besides having
developed food allergies, they are likely to suffer from an
infestation of the intestinal yeast/fungus, *Candida albicans*.
(see chapter 2). This may result in the development of hypersensitivity or allergy to any yeast found in the diet. The diagnosis of a yeast problem is not clearcut and is best made by

your doctor. Still, it is useful to know the signs associated with yeast-related problems and the sources of yeast in the diet.

Signs that your child's illness may be yeast-related include:[20]

- History of antibiotics.
- Sensitivity to tobacco smoke, perfumes, paint fumes, other odors.
- Fatigue, sluggishness, lethargy.
- Irritability, hyperactivity, inability to concentrate.
- Fungal infections of the mouth, skin, toe nails, or finger nails.
- Recurring digestive upset, gas, diarrhea.
- Symptoms aggravated by eating.
- Symptoms aggravated from antibiotics.
- Symptoms aggravated when in a moldy area.

Foods that aggravate yeast problems include:[21]

- Refined sugars.
- Anything containing malt (often added to cereals).
- Nuts (especially peanuts and nuts that are not fresh).
- Leftovers (mold grows quickly as foods begin to cool).
- Cheeses.
- Vitamins (especially B-vitamins unless labeled "yeast-free").
- Fruit juices (unless freshly prepared).
- Anything with baker's yeast or brewer's yeast listed on the label.

If your child appears to improve while on a diet free of offending foods, the first step is to keep him off the offenders.

While important, I believe this is not enough. Allergy and hypersensitivity develop for a reason. Keeping children off certain foods indefinitely is not an acceptable long-term solution (although some children may do well on this type of program). You will want to identify the underlying weaknesses that allow those allergies to develop and correct them. Allergy can be triggered by digestive problems, fatty acid deficiency, trace mineral deficiency, exposure to toxic substances, and numerous other factors. Some of the alternative treatments described in chapter 8 can often reduce the incidence of allergy significantly. For these reasons, the assistance of a health professional will likely be required.

Rotation Diets

A rotation diet refers to the practice of eating certain foods on a schedule. The schedule may consist of eating a food every other day, every five days, every seven days, or some variation. For instance, a child allergic to wheat may have trouble eating wheat every day, but may do well if wheat consumption is restricted to every fifth day. Rotation diets have value in several capacities. First, they can be used in instances where it is unclear which foods are causing problems. Some parents help to reduce illness in their children simply by feeding them on a rotation diet. Second, in cases where a child has multiple food allergies, complete elimination may be difficult and impractical. There also may be concerns about nutritional adequacy. In these instances, adopting a food rotation diet helps reduce her exposure to problem foods, while still providing adequate balance.

Finally, rotation diets can be used when reintroducing an offending food back into the diet. If your child has had recurrent earaches that have responded well to food allergy management, you will at some point want to attempt to reintroduce the food(s) back into her diet—after at least six to nine symptom-free months. (Children with a history of anaphylaxis related to food should see a doctor before making any dietary changes.) You first introduce the least offending food. Once you've determined that it produces no symptoms, add the next offending food. This is done over a period of a few days. Let's assume you find that all the problem foods now produce no symptoms. Adding them back on an everyday basis would be unwise. That might be the quickest way back to trouble. However, you can add them back on a rotation schedule.

For more information on rotation diets, see *Dr. Mandell's Five-Day Allergy Relief System*, by Marshall Mandell, M.D., and *Brain Allergies*, by Dr. William Philpott.

Homeopathic Medicine

Homeopathy is a comprehensive and effective form of medicine that works by stimulating the inherent recuperative abilities of the body. The word homeopathy is derived from the Greek words *homoios* meaning "similar" and *pathos*, which means "disease" or "suffering." Nearly 200 years ago, a German physician named Samuel Hahnemann observed that any plant, animal, or mineral substance ingested in excess caused a distinct pattern of symptoms. Through a series of exhaustive experiments and observations, Dr. Hahnemann found that these symptom patterns could be cured by ingesting a minute amount (microdose) of the same substance. This phenomenon of "like cures like" is what led Hahnemann to describe the "law of similars" which has become the fundamental pharmacologic principle of homeopathic medicine.

For example, arsenic is a known poison that causes certain types of fever and digestive disturbance. Homeopathic *Arsenicum* is used to treat fever and digestive disturbance. Overdose of the plant *Belladonna* results in flushed skin, swollen tonsils, high fever, and dilated pupils. Homeopathic *Belladonna* is successful at treating these same symptoms.

We're all familiar with the "law of similars" and the law of microdoses. Modern allergy practice is loosely based upon it. A child develops hay fever and seeks medical help. His doctor conducts allergy tests and recommends shots that contain minute amounts of the very items to which the child is allergic. However, there are few similarities between allergy shots and homeopathic medicines.

What makes homeopathic medicines different from their sometimes toxic counterparts? First, homeopathic medicines begin with a plant, animal, or mineral substance that is diluted sequentially 3 times, 200 times, or even 100,000 times or more. At these dilutions, none of the toxic effects of the original substance remain. It is at this level that homeopathic medicines become powerful healing tools. Another feature that distinguishes homeopathic medicines is the process of potentization through which a remedy must go. At each stage of dilution a homeopathic mixture must be vigorously shaken. This causes a form of physical activation. The combination of dilution and potentization is what makes homeopathic medicines effective.

The effects of potentized substances have been proven in the laboratory, and in studies with humans and animals. Penicillin, a well-known inhibitor of bacteria, has been shown to inhibit the growth of sensitive bacteria even when present in dilutions of 1:50,000,000 to 1:100,000,000.[22] In 1964, two researchers at the Pasteur Institute showed that mice could eliminate an endotoxin* when given only 1/10,000 of a microgram of the endotoxin.[23] DDVP, a powerful insecticide, is used in concentrated doses to kill locusts and other insect species. It is also highly toxic to humans and animals. A 1989 report showed that DDVP also exerts insecticidal effects at dilutions as high as 1:10,000,000.[24]

Numerous clinical trials have shown the value of homeopathic medicine in treating disease in humans. In a double-blind study of hay fever sufferers, published in the British

---

*Endotoxins are toxic substances contained within bacterial cells.

medical journal *Lancet*, patients given a 30c homeopathic dilution of 12 grass pollens experienced six times the improvement
as those given a placebo. Those under homeopathic care asked
for antihistamines only half as often as the placebo group.[25] A
recent controlled study showed that doctors obtained good
results using homeopathic *Pulsatilla* in the care of children
with acute otitis media.[26, 27]

Clinically, homeopaths report exceptional results managing both acute and chronic forms of otitis media. Acute otitis
media is more responsive to homeopathic home care. Chronic
otitis media often requires the expertise of a trained homeopath. However, acute episodes are common with chronic
otitis media, and the acute episodes can often be managed at
home with homeopathy. It is my opinion that homeopathic
medicine is among the quickest and safest forms of home care
available. More importantly, it is one of the most effective.

Potencies

There are two common systems of preparing homeopathic
remedies. In one system, one part of the starting material
(plant or mineral substance) is diluted to 99 parts liquid. This
system is known as the centesimal system—remedies are
given the designation "*c*." The other method uses a dilution of
one part medicine to 9 parts liquid—these are designated "*x*."
The number of times a remedy is sequentially diluted in one
of these ways is referred to as the dilution. A remedy diluted
one part to 99 parts, 6 times, is called a 6c remedy. A remedy
diluted one part to 9 parts, 6 times, is called a 6x remedy. For
practical purposes 6c and 6x are no different.

Potencies range from 1x (or 1c) to 1,000,000x (or
1,000,000c) and higher.

For home care, it is best to purchase remedies in either
the 6th (6c or 6x), 12th (12c or 12x), or 30th (30c or 30x)
potency. In general, 30th potencies are deeper and faster acting, but usually require a more accurate remedy selection.
Most home care prescribers achieve excellent results using

either the 6th or 12th potencies. Proper selection of remedy is more important than the potency chosen.

Dosage

For severe symptoms, the remedy you choose should be given four to six times per day. When symptoms are of a lesser degree, two to four doses daily until symptoms improve are all that is needed. Remedies can be purchased in both liquid and tablet form. Tablets are preferred for children since they are quite palatable. For small children, the tablets should be ground into a powder and given by mouth. The powder also can be mixed with a small amount of water and taken orally.

Remedies are given until there is an improvement in symptoms. Once you notice improvement, the remedy is discontinued. If symptoms resume after a short time, you can give the remedy again. (You may wish to try the next higher potency if this occurs.)

It is not unusual to see dramatic improvement after only one or two doses of a remedy. You can expect most to take longer. If you see no improvement within two or three days, you have probably chosen the wrong remedy. If this occurs, reexamine your child's symptoms and choose another remedy. If, after two or three attempts you're unsuccessful, there are probably other contributing factors.

Healing Crisis

Homeopaths have long recognized a phenomenon known as a healing crisis (also called an aggravation). Sometime soon after the first couple of doses, the child (or adult for that matter) may experience a brief aggravation of symptoms. This is a positive sign (although its absence is not negative) that indicates a deep-acting healing response is occurring. A healing crisis can be differentiated from a true worsening of a child's condition by noting the way in which the changes come about. In a healing crisis, the aggravation of symptoms is usually abrupt and occurs shortly after beginning a remedy. After a brief period of aggravation, the condition begins to improve noticeably. In contrast, when a condition is truly deteriorating, the symptoms may rapidly or slowly get worse, but they continue to decline.

The effects of homeopathic medicines can be profound. In chapter 1, I described the case of four-year-old Tiffany who responded exceptionally well to allergy management. As I related, she had tympanostomy tubes placed in both ears at two and a half years of age. The first tube fell out within seven months of its placement, but the other remained for over 18 months, which greatly concerned the surgeon. Tiffany had been scheduled for surgery for removal of the second tube. However, her parents were reluctant to have her anesthetized again. Two weeks before the surgery date, they asked if I had any suggestions. I recommended Tiffany take homeopathic *Merc dulc* daily for the next week. Within the week, she rejected the second tube. When she arrived at the hospital for her pre-surgical screening, the otolaryngologist told the parents that the tube was no longer in the eardrum and that the eardrum looked "quite good."

Children who don't extrude their tubes within a reasonable period are often constitutionally weak. In Tiffany's case, allergy management helped her earaches considerably, but did not restore her to full strength. The homeopathic medicine improved her constitutional strength sufficiently to reject the tube.

Antagonists

One peculiar aspect of homeopathic medicines is that they can be antidoted by several common substances. This antidoting effect can negate the useful effects of homeopathic medicines on the body. These substances should be avoided when using homeopathic medicines. They include products that contain camphor (some lip balms, Ben Gay, Vick's Vapo-rub, Heet, Campho-Phenique, Noxema), mint or menthol (Hall's cough drops, some toothpastes), and coffee. It is also helpful to avoid substances containing the oils of eucalyptus, rosemary, pennyroyal or other strongly aromatic herbs while taking homeopathic medicines. [28]

Single Remedies

Selecting the proper homeopathic remedy to care for an earache, while not always easy, is rather straightforward. It requires that you observe both the physical and mental signs displayed by your child and match them with the remedy that most closely relates to those signs. It is important not to over-look emotional, mental, or behavioral signs in your child. These are often the most useful in selecting the appropriate remedy.

Following the description of each remedy is a listing of what makes the child's symptoms worse and what makes them better. These are called *modalities* in homeopathic terminology. For instance, the child in need of the remedy *Hepar sulph* is better with warmth, and worse from cold and touch. Mod-alities are not listed for therapeutic purposes, although there is no doubt that keeping the *Hepar* child warm and avoiding touch will make her more comfortable. Modalities are listed to help guide you to the proper remedy selection. If the child above displays some signs indicating *Hepar sulph*, but is not bothered by touch or cold, chances are that a different remedy is needed.

The remedies most commonly used in home care situa-tions include: *Aconite, Belladonna, Chamomilla, Ferrum phos-phoricum, Hepar sulphuricum, Lycopodium, Mercurius, Plan-tago, Pulsatilla,* and *Silica*. It is important to note that a child need not display all the symptoms of a medicine for that medicine to be effective.

Aconite

This remedy is required when otitis media is caused by expo-sure to cold wind or a sudden change of temperature. The onset is usually rapid and accompanied by fever. Thirst is almost always present. The external ear is hot, red, painful, and swollen. Anxiety, fear, and restlessness are the most notable mental signs. These children are oversensitive to noise and touch. Unlike the *Belladonna* child, who is delirious and unaware of her surroundings, the *Aconite* child is very alert. The cheeks may be red, hot, flushed, or swollen. On rising, the face may become pale. At times, one cheek may be pale while the other is flushed. This remedy is usually only used in the first 24 hours of an earache that has come on rapidly. Beyond 24 hours, another remedy is usually indicated.

Symptoms are worse: from warmth, a warm room, and at night.

Symptoms are better: in open air.

Belladonna

Belladonna, like *Aconite*, is indicated when an earache comes on suddenly. In fact, *Belladonna* is the most commonly used remedy in the early stages of acute otitis media. The illness is usually associated with hot, red skin, flushed face, glaring eyes, restless sleep, and hypersensitivity of all senses. The throat is hot and dry with swollen tonsils. There is usually fever present, but the skin is dry. There is commonly no thirst. The ear, ear canal, and eardrum will often be bright red. Ear pain commonly extends down into the throat. *Belladonna* is associated with high fever that sets in abruptly with little warning. In some cases, there will be few symptoms other than earache and fever. The emotional symptoms are important with *Belladonna*. The child is almost unaware of what is going on around her. The acuteness of her senses may cause her to be agitated and furious, which may lead to outbursts of hitting or biting. These children may have fear of imaginary things, hallucinations and delirium. The pupils are dilated. *Belladonna* should be considered anytime there is intense pain.

Symptoms are worse: from touch, motion, noise, draft, light, odors, and lying on the painful side.

Symptoms are better: from sitting semi-erect.

Chamomilla

This is one of the most commonly used remedies in the care of otitis media. Children in need of *Chamomilla* are irritable and cross. They want something, but when given it are likely to throw it back at you. They are not easily consoled, but may feel better if carried around. They are impatient, and are intolerant of being spoken to, interrupted, or even looked at. If the child is mentally calm, they likely do not need *Chamomilla*. The *Chamomilla* child has bright red cheeks. At times, one cheek may be red while the other is pale. There is acute, stabbing ear pain that may drive the child frantic. Nasal mucus is clear, and discharge from the ear is not typical. The symptoms come on rapidly, although not as rapidly as with *Belladonna*.

Chamomilla is a commonly used remedy for the discomfort associated with teething. If a child is teething and her symptoms match the other symptoms of *Chamomilla* (especially the emotional signs), consider giving *Chamomilla*.

Symptoms are worse: from heat, open air, cold, wind, touch, eating, warmth of the bed, lying down, and at night.

Symptoms are better: from being rocked or carried, warm wet weather, and cold applications.

Ferrum phosphoricum

This is for the child whose earache comes on rapidly, but not as rapidly as with *Belladonna*. The child is feverish but not as severe as with *Belladonna*. The eardrum is red and bulging. *Ferrum phos* is often indicated after exposure to wet weather or when *Belladonna* fails to give relief.

Symptoms are worse: at night and from touch.

Symptoms are better: with cold applications.

Hepar Sulphuricum

Hepar is generally not used in the early stages of an earache. It is used when symptoms have progressed and pus has formed in the middle ear. There is frequently a nasal discharge that is at first watery, then becomes thick, yellow, and offensive. There is intense throbbing pain in the ear, accompanied by diminished hearing. These children are irritable and sensitive. Like the *Chamomilla* child, the *Hepar* child is cross and easily angered. They can be provoked to a tantrum with little effort. A hallmark of the *Hepar* child is oversensitivity to touch, cold, and pain. The cold sensitivity may be so great that even a hand or foot exposed from beneath the covers results in aggravation of symptoms.

Symptoms are worse: from dry cold winds, cold foods, touch, pressure, the slightest draft, exertion, or at night.

Symptoms are better: from warmth, extra clothing or covers, humidity, hot applications, and after eating.

Lycopodium

A characteristic of this remedy is symptoms that are on or begin on the right side. There may be a humming and roaring sensation in the ear, with diminished hearing. A thick, yellow, offensive discharge is common. The nose is stopped up. *Lycopodium* is especially indicated in children with digestive complaints such as gas and bloating. These children are thin and weak. They often have cold hands and feet. The *Lycopodium* child is fearful, apprehensive, and afraid to be alone. They are averse to taking on new things. They can be headstrong and scornful when sick. This is a remedy that may be used at any stage of an earache.

Symptoms are worse: from lying on the right side, heat or a warm room, hot air, cold food or drink, eating, and from 4 to 8 p.m.

Symptoms are better: from warm food and drink, being uncovered, motion, cool or open air, and after midnight.

Mercurius

Mercurius is indicated when there is pus formation and is often used in more chronic cases of otitis media. The nasal discharge is yellow-green and offensive (as are all body secretions in these children). There is profuse, offensive perspiration.

Lymph nodes are typically swollen. There is great thirst. The skin is almost constantly moist. If the skin is consistently dry, *Mercurius* is not the remedy. Increased salivation, bad breath and puffiness of the tongue are general *Mercurius* symptoms.

The child in need of *Mercurius* is often described as a human "thermometer" because she is acutely sensitive to heat, cold, and most all environmental influences. *Mercurius* children are weak and may tire at the slightest exertion. There is sometimes muscular trembling. These children seem to display a loss of will-power.

Symptoms are worse: from damp, cold, rainy weather, heat, sweating, motion, exertion, open air, lying on the right side, in a warm bed or warm room, and at night.

Symptoms are better: in moderate temperatures.

Plantago major

Plantago major is needed when ear pain is associated with teething or toothache. The pain often goes from one ear to the other through the head. Intolerance to noise is common. There is a watery, yellowish nasal discharge.

Pulsatilla

This is one of the most frequently used remedies in otitis media and is suitable for almost all types of ear pain. Children needing *Pulsatilla* tend to be gentle, weepy, sensitive, and love to be held. They want attention and are easily consoled by a sympathetic response. *Pulsatilla* children are sometimes described as moody because they can be happy one moment and profoundly sad the next. They often feel sorry for themselves and lament their plight during illness.

Their cheeks are pale. They feel better when in open, fresh air. There is a thick, bland, yellowish-green nasal discharge. The eardrum is swollen and red, with fluid. If the ear is draining, the discharge is usually thick and yellowish-green. The ear is swollen, red, and hot, and there is deep itching in it. The pain often goes through the whole side of the face.

There may be a stopped sensation in the ear. A dry or loose cough can be present. Symptoms often come on gradually and frequently follow a cold. The child may be feverish, but show a surprising absence of thirst.

Symptoms are worse: from heat, lying down, exertion, after eating, toward evening, and in a warm room.

Symptoms are better: from motion, cold applications, cold food and drink, and in open air.

Silica

Children in need of *Silica* are likely to experience discharge from the ear. They are sensitive and anxious. *Silica* is often indicated when a cold or bronchial condition is long-standing or slow to respond. Symptoms are severe. There is often roaring in the ears, and the child is sensitive to noise. The *Silica* child is cold, chilly, and wants plenty of warm clothing. He hates drafts, and his hands and feet are icy cold. There is offensive sweat on the hands, feet, and armpits. *Silica* is the remedy most often indicated when there is pain behind the ear on the mastoid process. (See also *Hepar sulph.*)

Mentally these children are yielding, faint-hearted, and anxious. They are nervous, excitable, and sensitive, but can be obstinate. *Silica* children tend to be weak and easily exhausted.

Symptoms are worse: from cold, open air, winter, damp weather, cold food or drink, lying on the painful side, eating, and in morning.

Symptoms are better: from warmth.

It is not always easy to decide which homeopathic medicine your child might need. Often the choice can be narrowed down to two or three medicines, but the final selection can be difficult. To make this process easier, a series of flow charts has been designed by Dr. Stephen Messer. These charts can be found in chapter 8 under Homeopathic Medicine. The figures labeled Otitis Media Without Effusion and Acute Otitis Media are those most likely to be useful in home care. Recognize that proper use of these charts depends upon making a specific diagnosis of the middle ear condition.

Ear Drops

Ear drops are discussed in the section on botanical medicine, but one excellent homeopathic eardrop formula deserves mention here. **Traumeel** is a patent formula made by Biological Homeopathic Industries. David Riley, M.D., reports that Traumeel applied topically can provide substantial relief when ear pain strikes. It can be purchased in liquid form. To apply this formula, warm several drops on a teaspoon, then place 3 drops in each ear and cover with cotton. (This is not for use in an ear where you see drainage.)

Traumeel consists of:*

Arnica D2	*Calendula* D2
Hamamelis D2	*Millefolium* D3
Belladonna D4	*Aconitum* D3
Hepar sulfuris D5	*Mercuris solubilis Hahnemanni* D8
Chamomilla D3	*Symphytum* D3
Bellis perennis D2	*Echinacea angustifolia* D2
Echinacea purpurea D2	*Hypericum* D2

Colds and Nasal Congestion

Homeopathic medicine is very effective at treating the symptoms of colds, sinus, and nasal congestion that often precede otitis media. If your child is prone to earaches, any cold or sinus problem should be managed homeopathically. The appropriate remedies are discussed in chapter 7.

For more information on homeopathic medicine, I suggest you read the books *Homeopathy: Medicine for the Twenty-first Century*, by Dana Ullman, M.P.H., and *Everybody's Guide to Homeopathic Medicines*, by Stephen Cummings, F.N.P, and Dana Ullman, M.P.H.

---

*The "D" designation is equivalent to the "x" discussed above.

Rather than simply purchasing individual remedies, I recommend that parents purchase a homeopathic remedy kit. Kits come in all sizes, ranging from those that contain 10 remedies all the way up to 50. Having a variety of remedies at your disposal will allow you to administer home care for many common childhood complaints including colic, upset stomach, colds, bumps, bruises, and more.

To order books and remedies, see the resource section of this book.

Spinal Manipulation

The use of manipulation of the vertebrae and other joints of the body has been a part of medical systems throughout recorded history. The Chinese have used manipulation for more than two thousand years as an integral part of their medical system. During the time of Hippocrates, manipulation of the vertebrae was used to treat a variety of disorders, especially those of a musculoskeletal origin. Manipulation of the vertebrae (and other joints) has seen a rapid rebirth in contemporary Western medicine through the practice of chiropractic and osteopathy. The body of evidence of the therapeutic value of manipulation is growing steadily.

When biomechanical problems of the upper spine contribute to otitis media, correction of these problems becomes an integral part of treatment. Dr. Gottfried Gutmann makes three important points on biomechanical problems, manipulation, and recurrent infections. He concludes that: 1) blocked nerve impulses at the atlas [first cervical vertebrae] contribute to lower resistance to infections of the ear, nose and throat, 2) chiropractic and radiological examinations are "of decisive importance" for diagnosis of the syndrome, and 3) "chiropractic can often bring about amazingly successful results, because the therapy is a causal one."[29, 30]

Manipulation is discussed here not because it is a method of home care, but to show its place in the overall scheme of how otitis media must be viewed from a treatment perspective. In cases of biomechanical problems that require manipulation, a doctor of chiropractic or osteopathy must be consulted. See chapter 8 for a more detailed discussion of manipulation.

Acupressure

The practice of Chinese medicine traditionally includes diet, exercise, manipulation, massage, meditation, bone-setting, herbs and acupuncture. The term acupuncture describes one of many methods of stimulating various locations on the body known as acupoints. Acupressure is another common means of stimulating these points.

Over the years, the Chinese have discovered that specific acupoints have specific functions. The stimulation of these points causes predictable changes to occur throughout the body.

For example, the point Large Intestine 4 is said to eliminate pathogenic wind from the head and face. Crudely translated, pathogenic wind refers to viral influences. (The Chinese lacked knowledge of viruses as we know them today, but their clinical descriptions are profoundly accurate.) In practice, Large Intestine 4 (LI-4) has a significant effect on symptoms of headache, toothache, sore throat, fever, earache, and the common cold. Thus, the point LI-4 would be stimulated in certain types of earaches.

The point San Jiao 5 (SJ-5, or TH-5) is known to expel wind (thus having an influence on what we would call viral syndromes) and regulate the San Jiao channel. The San Jiao channel refers to a meridian, or pathway, through which energy travels. The San Jiao channel circles the ear and sends a branch through the ear. Regulation of this channel is important in correcting the problems that exist during an ear infection. In actual practice, treating San Jiao 5 can have remarkable effects on the progress of otitis media. I've observed acute inflammatory middle ear problems resolve fully in just 24 hours using this and one other point.

What if an earache occurs with high fever, signs of heat, and inflammation that does not subside? In Chinese medicine this is called pathogenic wind-heat. This description, while foreign to Westerners, tells the acupuncturist that points must be used that will dissipate or clear this wind-heat. One point which serves this purpose is called Du-14. Clinically, this point is used in febrile illnesses, the common cold, cough, asthma, and earache. Du-14 is used with other pertinent acupoints to correct the underlying syndrome that has manifested as middle ear inflammation. In the Chinese system of medicine, there are points that cover the whole range of therapeutic application. This makes Chinese medicine an extremely useful and versatile system of healing.

In Chinese medicine, illness is not viewed as a cause and effect phenomenon. The Chinese view illness as an expression of patterns of disharmony. The acupuncturist makes his diagnosis based upon a careful physical examination of the patient. Questions about the child's behavior, habits, and symptomatology are asked. This information is used to identify the pattern involved. Once the pattern has been identified, the acupuncturist selects the points (usually only 2-4 points with children) that would be most successful in correcting the underlying disharmony. The points are then stimulated for a brief period using needles, pressure, or any number of other methods employed today. It is important to note that the results of acupuncture are enhanced by the concurrent use of botanical medicine.

Acupressure for Earaches

You obviously won't be doing acupuncture at home, but you can use acupressure, which is often very effective at alleviating the symptoms of earache. Stimulating acupoints with pressure is useful because it can influence lymph drainage, reduce pain, and sometimes encourage removal of fluid from the middle ear.

To treat the acupoints, have your child lie down comfortably on the bed. First, locate all of the points you will be treating. (See figure 11.) You'll notice that some points are near the ear while others are as far away as the foot. In this treatment, you begin with the point furthest from the ear. Once you have stimulated it, you go to the next closest, and so on.

Stimulation of the point is achieved by placing your thumb over it and placing slight to moderate pressure in a gentle massaging motion. Continue this for one minute. If the pressure you are using causes pain, ease up a little. As you get to the points closest to the ear, you may find they are so tender that your child will not let you touch them. If this is the case, avoid these points.

The points used in the home care of earaches, in order of first treated to last are:

1. GB-41	5. TH-5
2. KI-7	6. GB-20
3. KI-3	7. TH-17 (gently)
4. LI-4	8. GB-2

This acupressure treatment can be done two to three times per day.

Clearing Lymphatic Congestion

Another useful method that can be employed at home when a case of otitis media occurs is the "Lymphatic Flush," used to enhance the function of the tonsils and adenoids.

The tonsils and adenoids are part of the lymphatic system. Connecting these and other lymph structures, including lymph nodes, is a large network of lymphatic vessels. It is the job of the lymphatic vessels to transport waste products throughout the body to be eliminated. They also serve as a pathway for the movement of white blood cells to the site of infection.

At times, flow through the lymphatic vessels of the head and neck is reduced due to swelling, inflammation, mechanical obstruction, infection, allergy, and so on. If the lymphatic ves-

Figure 11
Acupoints Used in Otitis Media

sels don't drain, the tonsils and adenoids cannot eliminate waste products and thus become more swollen. This leads to obstruction of the eustachian tube, preventing normal drainage. Impaired drainage results in fluid accumulation in the middle ear and aggravation of ear pain.

The lymphatic flush technique can be done at home to enhance drainage and improve the environment around the eustachian tube. This often greatly enhances the healing of the middle ear. I've recommended this to parents for years. The results are exceptional.

The Lymphatic Flush (see figure 12)

1. Have your child lie down on his back, with his head slightly elevated.

2. Apply a generous helping of unscented hand lotion to your hands. Make sure that your hands and the lotion are warm.

3. Gently rub the lotion up and down the front and sides of your child's neck. This will spread the lotion and also get your child accustomed to your touch. Remember, he is in pain so proceed slowly.

4. The area you're treating lies along the large muscle which is located on the front and side of the neck (called the sternocleidomastoid). Using a broad hand contact, and beginning about one inch up from the collarbone on each side (the dimensions will vary depending upon the age and size of the child), stroke your hand downward in the direction of the collarbone. Use moderate pressure and repeat five or six times.

5. Place your hands two inches up from the collarbone and stroke downward five or six times.

6. Next, place your hands one inch higher than the previous time and stroke downward five or six times.

Figure 12-a
Lymph Nodes of the Head and Neck

Figure 12-b
Lymphatic Flush Technique

7. Repeat this until your hands are up at the tonsils. At this point, you will be making long strokes from the tonsils downward.

The purpose of this exercise is to encourage fluid to drain away from the tonsils, thus reducing the amount of congestion in that area. You begin at the bottom because it is necessary to clear an area of stagnant lymph fluid. Once the lower lymph vessels are open, it will be easier to move the above fluid downward. This technique can provide substantial relief to an ailing child.

Spinal Massage

The spinal massage is done by having your child lie down on the bed on his belly. It can be done with your child's shirt on or off, depending on which is more comfortable to him. I prefer to stimulate the bare skin. If you do this, use unscented lotion, and make sure your hands and the room are warm enough.

With your child on his belly, begin in the small of the back and massage along both sides of the spine, working your way upward as you go. Work slowly and gently, spending about 30 seconds at each level. Continue until you reach the base of the skull. The entire exercise should take roughly ten minutes.

There are three main reasons for doing this procedure. First, treatment of this area stimulates drainage of some of the lymphatic vessels affecting the lungs. Second, the autonomic nervous system can be influenced. (This part of the nervous system controls automatic functions such as secretion of mucus.) And third, the acupuncture association points are stimulated. (See figure 13.) All along the spinal column lie acupuncture points that associate with each major organ system. General stimulation of these points can enhance the integrated functions of the body during illness.

Children love to be massaged. You will be amazed at how

Figure 13
Association Points of Acupuncture

Reprinted from *Applied Kinesiology Synopsis*, Systems DC, Pueblo, Colorado, Copyright 1988, with permission.

much this can improve your child's well-being and enhance his recovery.

Acupressure for Colds and Nasal Congestion

The longer the nasal cavity remains congested, the greater the likelihood of congestion developing in the middle ear. A simple acupressure treatment can often aid in reducing nasal congestion. (Obviously if other factors exist, you will have to identify these as well.)

1. Have your child lie down on his back with his head slightly elevated. You should be seated at his head.
2. Using the pads of your fingers, gently massage the points listed in figure 14.
3. Spend about 45 seconds treating each point. The entire treatment should take about 7 minutes.

The points used in the treatment of colds and nasal congestion include:

1. DU-16	5. LI-20
2. DU-20	6. BL-4
3. BL-12	7. LU-7
4. GB-20	

Botanical Medicine

The use of plants to treat disease is perhaps the oldest form of medicine known. Today, both botanical medicine and allopathic medicine depend heavily upon the same plants used centuries ago. Nearly 70 percent of today's patent drugs are manufactured using knowledge of plant substances, and 25 percent have substances extracted directly from plants. For example, the drug Ephedra is used widely in the West to treat respiratory conditions. This drug is derived from the Chinese plant known as Ma Huang, or *Ephedra sinica*. The use of Ma Huang to treat respiratory conditions was documented in Chinese medical literature centuries ago.

For hundreds of years herbalists treated colds, inflammation, and pain by having patients chew on the bark of black willow, or meadowsweet. Today we take it in the form more

Figure 14
Acupoints for Colds and Nasal Congestion

commonly known as aspirin, the name of which is derived
from the old botanical name of meadowsweet, Spirea.[31]

The clinical results obtained in the skilled practice of
botanical medicine worldwide are impressive. Clinical and laboratory studies in the West continue to elucidate the specific
actions of plant substances. For instance, St. John's Wort (*Hyper-
icum triquetrifolium*) has been shown to interfere with viral
infection and replication.[32] Constituents found in the *shitake*
mushroom (*Lentinus edodes*) affect viruses indirectly by
enhancing T and B lymphocyte function and stimulating natural killer cells. This plant also has anti-tumor activity.[33]

The common milk thistle (*Silybum marianum*) contains,
as its chief active ingredient, a compound called silymarin,
which is reputed to be one of the most potent liver-protecting
substances known. Silymarins are powerful antioxidants. This
compound stimulates the production of new liver cells to
replace damaged cells. Studies in Finland, Russia, and Europe
have shown this healing effect to occur in people with sus-
tained liver damage due to diabetes, alcohol, drugs, environmental toxins, and viruses.[34]

Given the rich history of botanical medicine and the emerging scientific confirmation of its value, it is no surprise that
botanical medicine has a role to play in the management of
childhood otitis media. Recently, Ikeda and Takasaka reported
a study using Kampo medicine to treat secretory otitis media.
Kampo medicine, or *Sairei-to*,* as it's called in Japan, consists
of eight different herbs. This investigation was based on evidence that Kampo medicine is effective in resolving conditions
that exhibit inflammatory and immunological reactions. An
advantage of using Kampo medicine is that it causes few

Sairei-to consists of the herbs *Bupleurum falcatum*, *Alisma
orientale*, *Pinellia ternata*, *Scutellaria baicalensis*, *Zizyphus jujuba*,
Panax ginseng, *Cinnamomum cassia*, and *Zingiber officinale*.

adverse effects even in long-term treatment—a desirable feature where children are concerned. At the completion of this four-week trial, the authors concluded that "Kampo medicine may resolve the inflammation and immune response associated with secretory otitis media."[35]

While botanical medicine can be helpful in managing otitis media, prescribing herbal combinations is a complex process. There are numerous different syndromes in otitis media, each of which requires different herbal formulas. Thus, for home care purposes, I've listed only those that 1) are used as ear drops to relieve pain, 2) build energy in constitutionally weak children, and 3) act as general immune stimulants.

Ear Drops

Ear drops are not generally known to cure earaches, but they can provide what most parents and children are after—relief of symptoms. The most effective herbs used as drops include:

- *Plantago major* tincture.
- *Pennywort* tincture.
- *Mullein* oil.
- *Chamomile* infusion.
- *Olive* oil.
- The Three Yellows (see chapter 8).

It's only necessary to use one of the above at any given time. I've listed several because you may find that one does not work for your child. In such a case, choose another on the list. I've found *Plantago major* to be very effective, especially when the earaches are associated with teething problems. Martha Benedict, an acupuncturist in Santa Cruz, California, claims exceptional results using the three yellows.[36]

The herb solution should be heated slightly by placing a

few drops on a spoon and warming it for a few seconds with a match from underneath. Using a dropper, which is usually provided with the herbal mixture, withdraw the herb from the spoon and test a drop on the inside of your wrist to make sure it is not too warm. Next, place three drops in the affected ear and cover with a piece of cotton. The application should be repeated three times per day during the course of the earache. You may wish to use the same piece of cotton for a day or two, since it will be saturated and less likely to absorb the herb the next time you use it in the ear. Eardrops should not be used when there is fluid draining out of the middle ear.

Most of the above herbs are available at health food stores or can be ordered from the companies listed in the resource section.

Herbal Teas

Herbal teas can be used to reduce mucous congestion and build energy in a weakened or sick child.

For children with excessive mucus production, you can make a tea that consists of water, one-eighth teaspoon of raw honey, a few drops of brandy, and fresh ground ginger root, cinnamon, or cayenne.

Nose Drops

Clearing the nasal passages can sometimes help speed recovery of the middle ear. In addition, clear nasal passages allow the child to breathe more easily, which goes a long way toward ensuring a much-needed night's sleep for both you and your child.

One type of nose drop that occasionally proves helpful is a simple saltwater solution. This can be made by placing one teaspoon of table salt in a quart of warm water.

A nose drop that works exceptionally well is a mixture of fennelated Irish moss. Place one drop in the child's right nostril, then one in the left. Repeat until four drops have been placed in each nostril. At the time the first drop is placed, your child may notice a slight stinging sensation that quickly goes away once the second drop is applied and the Irish moss begins to do its work. The nose drops should be used four times a day during the active phase of an earache.

General Immune Stimulants

The most common botanical used in the West to enhance immune function is *Echinacea*. There have been more than 200 laboratory and clinical studies on the physiological effects of this herb. *Echinacea* has been shown to be anti-viral, anti-bacterial, and anti-fungal. Its use as a general immune tonic is widely known. Up to about 1930 and prior to the discovery of sulfa drugs, *Echinacea* was used regularly by physicians throughout the United States.[37]

Echinacea is usually purchased in tincture form. Five drops in a small glass of water can be given orally three times daily to a child over two. Under two years, give three drops three times daily.

Nutrition

Nutritional home care for earaches is a somewhat new area, and much remains to be learned. Still, there are certain fundamental approaches that can be used, based upon what we know about nutrition and inflammation, and nutrition and immune function.

Listed below are some nutrients that are useful in times of earache. I do not advise that all the items listed below be given in separate tablets. The list is provided as a guideline to suggest the nutrients that should be included in a multivitamin. Supplements such as evening primrose oil, flax oil, bifidus, acidophilus, and Inflavonoid are given separately.

A child who suffers from either acute or chronic earaches can be given:

ages 1–3	ages 4 and up
1 tsp. flax oil	2 tsp. flax oil
300–500 mg vitamin C	500–1,000 mg vitamin C
5–10 mg of zinc*	10 mg zinc*
Vitamin A 5,000 IU/day	Vitamin A 5,000 IU/day
Beta carotene 5,000 IU/day	Beta carotene 5,000 IU/day
Children's B-complex 1/day	Children's B-complex 2/day
Bifidus 2 tsp. per day (to age 7)	Acidophilus (age 7 & over) 2 Tbsp.
Inflavonoid 2 tablets/day	Inflavonoid 3 tablets/day
Vitamin E 25–50 IU/day	Vitamin E 50 IU/day
Magnesium 50 mg/day	Magnesium 50 mg/day

If a child is unresponsive to the above program you may wish to add evening primrose oil, 2 perles/day** for a child under three years of age and 3 perles/day for a child over 3.

Zinc and vitamin C can often be given together in a lozenge that is now available commercially. A child who chews these lozenges should have his teeth brushed afterward since ascorbic acid can be harmful to the enamel after prolonged contact with the teeth. Additional beta-carotene can be obtained by eating more orange and yellow vegetables such as carrots and squash. Vitamin A has a separate but important immune potentiating effect. It can be obtained from cod liver oil (which also contains omega-3 fatty acids).

Bifidobacteria are not found in any food products and

---

*Make sure the supplement contains about 3 micrograms of copper to balance with zinc. Do not give more zinc in hopes that more will stimulate the immune system better. Excess zinc inhibits immune function.

**Do not give perles to children under four or five. Break the perles open, and express the oil. Give the oil to your child by mouth or add it to juice, formula, or food. The proper dosage for children is one perle per year of age per day, up to six perles per day.

therefore must be purchased as a supplement (see discussion of acidophilus and bifidus). During an earache, avoid feeding your child sugar in any form—this includes fruit juice. A study at Loma Linda School of Medicine showed that fructose, sucrose, honey, or orange juice all significantly decreased the capacity of neutrophils (a white blood cell) to engulf bacteria. Children who are ill often don't feel like eating, and it's a good idea to follow their lead. During any type of infection or inflammation, the need for liquids increases so be sure to provide plenty of fluids.

Inflavonoid is a product that contains bioflavonoids (including curcumin) in concentrated amounts. Bioflavonoids are necessary to augment the function of vitamin C. They have a role in stimulating immune function. What is most impressive about bioflavonoids is that they block the inflammatory process by interfering with the enzymes that release inflammatory prostaglandins. However, unlike anti-inflammatory drugs such as acetaminophen, bioflavonoids do not block the enzyme needed for the body's own anti-inflammatory system. (See chapter 8 for more details.) To give inflavonoid to a child, I generally recommend breaking the tablet into a powder. This is preferable for all vitamin tablets.

Iron is necessary for fighting infection. Yet, excess iron can cause a variety of problems including immune suppression. I don't recommend that anyone take additional iron unless directed by their doctor. Doctors prescribing iron to patients should have good clinical or laboratory evidence of the need for iron before prescribing it. The best way for a child to obtain iron is from food. Nuts, blackstrap molasses, and dark turkey meat are good sources of iron. Iron absorption is enhanced when iron is taken with vitamin C-containing foods.

Since fatty acid imbalance plays such a large role in illness, it is important that you recognize the signs that may indicate fatty acid deficiency. If obvious signs of fatty acid deficiency exist you should take immediate steps to correct this through modifying your child's fat intake. It may be necessary to consult a practitioner knowledgeable in nutrition. The signs of fatty acid imbalance include:

- Follicular hyperkeratosis (so-called "chicken skin" on the upper arms—this also may suggest beta-carotene insufficiency).
- Dandruff on scalp.
- Hair that is dry and unmanageable.
- Areas of leukoplakia.
- Nails that are brittle, fray easily, or won't grow.
- Areas of "alligator skin" (anywhere on the body).
- Patches of pale, lusterless skin on the cheeks.
- Dry ear wax or excessive production of ear wax.
- Allergies.
- Excessive thirst.
- Hyperactivity (ADD).

The Importance of Intestinal Bacteria

Before birth, the fetal intestinal tract is sterile, i.e., it contains no bacteria. The intestinal bacteria arrive in the newborn as a result of transit through the birth canal, during which time the child is exposed to the mother's fecal and vaginal bacteria. Following this, the child is exposed to microbes from the skin, the environment, and food. This is nature's way of ensuring that the infant digestive tract contains the organisms needed to function properly. The intestinal bacteria outnumber the human cells in the entire body.

The most common bacteria in the infant digestive tract are *Bifidobacterium bifidus*, *Lactobacillus acidophilus* and *Escherichia coli*. *Bifidobacteria* account for about 99 percent of the intestinal bacteria in breastfed infants. Bottle-fed infants have far lower fecal levels of *Bifidobacteria*. After the child has been weaned, the number of *Bifidobacteria* decline rapidly. Meanwhile, *E. coli* and *L. acidophilus* increase in number until *E. coli* predominates.

Each of these bacteria perform necessary functions in the child's intestinal tract. *B. bifidus* and *L. acidophilus* possess the following beneficial functions:

- Allow for an increased number of lymphocytes and larger lymph nodes.

- Increase the number of plasma cells and serum immunoglobulins.

- Contribute to increased phagocytic activity in macrophages. The macrophages of germ-free animals digest bacteria more slowly, suggesting that the gut microbes play a role in macrophage activity.[38]

- Produce organic acids and hydrogen peroxide which kill invading microbes, thereby protecting the body against infection from food-or water-borne pathogens.[39]

- Synthesize important B-vitamins such as niacin, pantothenic acid, pyridoxine, biotin, and folic acid.[40]

- Digest lactose and other dietary components, and play a role in the digestion and assimilation of milk.[41]

- Allow for better utilization of nutrients from food. Germ-free animals (lacking intestinal bacteria) experience far more pronounced symptoms if their diet is deficient in nutrients than if the gut flora is intact.[42]

- Encourage more efficient weight gain.[43]

- Participate in detoxification of some toxic compounds that enter the body via food or water, thus protecting us from a toxic environment.[44]

- Inhibit certain types of tumor growth.[45]

- Prevent the fungus *Candida albicans* from forming invasive germ-tubes.[46]

- Inhibit the growth of *C. albicans* in both the digestive tract and vagina. *Candida albicans* is the organism present in vaginal yeast infections and oral thrush.[47]

- Protect against many microbial pathogens such as *Salmonella*, *Shigella*, and virulent strains of *E. coli*.

- Poduce organic acids that stimulate intestinal peristalsis, which in turn removes invading pathogens from the intestinal tract. (Peristalsis refers to the action of the intestinal muscles that moves the contents of the intestines forward.)

- Work in concert with the host immunological system (e.g., IgA).

In chapter 2, I said that antibiotics exert a pronounced adverse effect on the beneficial bacteria in the intestinal tract. You can see from the information above that the function of these bacteria is extremely important to the health of your child. Therefore, when antibiotics are being or have been used, it is important to reestablish these helpful bacteria in large numbers. This is accomplished by feeding the bacteria in some form to your child.

Supplementation of the diet with bacterial cultures has been used for centuries, most commonly as yogurt. Yogurt contains two main species of bacteria—*Streptococcus thermophilus* and *Lactobacillus bulgaricus*. *L. bulgaricus*, like *acidophilus*, is an acid-forming bacteria that digests lactose. It also inhibits harmful bacteria and parasites. This is one reason that consuming yogurt is associated with so many benefits. However, the bacteria found in yogurt, while helpful, are unable to attach to the intestinal wall, rendering them unable to establish a permanent colony. Because of this, the healing effects of yogurt are short-lived.

In contrast, *L. acidophilus* can become a permanent resident of the intestine by attaching tenaciously to the intestinal wall. In doing so, it prevents the attachment of many harmful organisms such as *Candida albicans* and *Giardia lamblia*. Unfortunately, any *L. acidophilus* added to yogurt is inhibited by *L. bulgaricus*, so simply adding *acidophilus* to yogurt is not a solution.*

The best long-term benefit is to be derived from *L. acidophilus* in children over seven, and *B. bifidus* in children under seven. Neither *L. acidophilus* nor *B. bifidus* are found naturally in foods. They are either obtained in supplement form or added to dairy products.

Who Might Need *Acidophilus* or *Bifidus* Supplements?

- Children with a history of oral thrush.

- Children with a history of diarrhea, constipation, or colic.

- Children known to have or suspected of having food allergies.

- Children with skin conditions such as eczema.

- Children believed to suffer from intestinal candidiasis.

- Infants born to a mother with a history of vaginal candidiasis.

- Hyperactive children where the hyperactivity appears to be associated with food allergy/sensitivity or digestive disturbance.

- Children with a history of antibiotic therapy.

- Children about to undergo antibiotic therapy.

- Children who have been bottlefed from birth or weaned before three months. All bottlefed children should receive bifidus daily.

---

*Yogurt is still an excellent food and can be used with great benefit provided your child is not sensitive to it. The point is that acidophilus or bifidus supplements yield better long-term results.

- Children who have had solid foods introduced before three months of age.

- Children born by C-section.

- Children with recurrent tonsillitis.

- Children with recurrent otitis media.

- Children with a recent history of intestinal viral infection. (Enteric viruses generally reduce the fecal levels of acid-forming bacteria to near zero.)

- Children with known parasitic infections such as *Giardia lamblia* or *Entamoeba histolytica*.

How Do I Find a Quality *Acidophilus* or *Bifidus* Supplement?

Here are some guidelines that will be helpful in determining which *acidophilus* or *bifidus* supplement to buy.

1. Purchase a powdered product that is *not* stored in capsules. Capsules absorb moisture, which typically shortens the shelf-life and reduces the number of viable organisms. Recently, some companies have begun to market packets of *acidophilus* and *bifidus*. This is the best method of preserving the maximum number of viable organisms. (See Metagenics and Nutrition Dynamics in appendix.)

2. These organisms are temperature-sensitive and must be refrigerated at all times. If you purchase it off the shelf (unrefrigerated), it is going to be less effective. Some companies will ship it in refrigerated containers upon request.

3. The number of viable organisms is important. Look for a product that specifically states the number of viable organisms. It should contain at least 1 billion or more. The label also should state the identifiable strain of organism since most of the research has been done on

strains DDS1 and NCFM. Other strains have not been as thoroughly tested for effectiveness.

4. *Bifidus* and *acidophilus* supplements (if used in the same program) are best taken at different times of the day.

5. Enteric coating of *acidophilus* or *bifidus* is an unnecessary process and serves only to reduce the number of viable organisms in the product. *Acidophilus* and *bifidus* are acid-loving organisms. Therefore, the environment of the stomach should not bother them appreciably unless the product contains a strain that is less hearty— something you're trying to avoid. Another problem with enteric coating is you can never predict if the coating will break down in time to insure maximum release of the organisms.

6. *Acidophilus* and *bifidus* should be purchased in a dairy base. Many companies now market *acidophilus* and *bifidus* supplements that are grown on a vegetable base for supposed use in people who are allergic to dairy. The most viable strains of acidophilus are only able to live on a dairy substrate. Moreover, calcium is needed by the microbes to attach to the intestinal wall and colonize. Without calcium, they do not attach so the benefits are short-lived.

   When these products are made, the organisms are first grown on milk solids. The milk solids are then filtered off, leaving only a small amount of the original substrate, thus minimizing the likelihood that a dairy-allergic individual would react. For individuals who do react adversely to a milk-based *acidophilus* or *bifidus*, a small dose should be used to begin, gradually building up to the standard dose. If this still does not work, a non-dairy product should be considered.

7. Sweet *acidophilus* milk contains living *acidophilus*, but in most cases, it is *Lactobacillus bulgaricus*—hearty,

but it doesn't colonize the intestinal tract. In addition, the numbers are considerably lower than in a high-quality supplement, making the milk unsuitable in a treatment program.

Sweet *acidophilus* milk would be acceptable as part of a maintenance program once reinoculation has been established (provided an allergy to casein does not exist).

8. If your child is under age seven, you want to use *bifidus*. If for some reason you have difficulty obtaining a *bifidus* supplement, by all means use acidophilus—it will still work wonders.

Dosage and Recommendations

1. ¼ teaspoon in ¼ glass of lukewarm water is frequently used to initiate therapy.

2. Dosage is often increased to ½ or 1 full teaspoon one to three times daily.

3. Take during mid-meal.

4. *Bifidus* is the recommended supplement for children under seven years.

5. *Bifidus* in conjunction with *acidophilus* enhances results. (*Bifidus* and *acidophilus* should be given at alternating times to avoid competitive inhibition.)

6. When given concurrently with an antibiotic, *bifidus* is best given at times between the antibiotic. When sulfa drugs are used, the spacing should be two to three hours.[48]

7. Obtain a high-quality product—this is essential!

Note: If adverse reactions occur, they are usually due to one or more of the following:

1. Herxheimer reaction. This occurs when organisms are killed abruptly, resulting in a release of the toxic contents within their cell membranes.

2. Inferior product.

3. Casein or lactose intolerance.

Putting It Together

In this chapter I've described a number of home care treatments that work well. Obviously, you will not be using all of these on your child. So here are some basic guidelines that will help you decide how to proceed.

1. Approach your child's problem as though it is related to food or airborne allergies until proven otherwise (Food allergies will likely be more common.) This means following the guidelines in the section on allergies. Remove dairy products temporarily and watch for improvement in your child's health. If allergies exist, remove the offenders from your child's diet or environment to the best of your ability. Adopt a strategy of rotation. Don't feed the same foods every day.

2. Assume there are nutritional needs that are not being met. This is especially true with essential fatty acids. Give essential fatty acids and other nutrients in the amounts listed.

3. Avoid known antagonists to good health including trans fatty acids, sugar, refined foods, and toxic metals. Reduce your child's intake of fruit juices, especially cold juices. When you give juice make sure it is fresh squeezed, not from concentrate. Follow the guidelines in chapter 7 that apply to your situation.

4. Choose a homeopathic medicine based on the symptoms of your child and the guidelines listed in the above section on homeopathy.

5. Use ear drops, nose drops, or acupressure to make your child more comfortable.

6. Give a *bifidus* supplement if your child falls into any of the categories listed in "Who Might Need *Acidophilus* or *Bifidus* Supplements?"

7. Take your child to the doctor if her condition does not respond within a reasonable amount of time. (See guidelines at the beginning of this chapter.)

Chapter 7

Preventing Ear Infections in Your Child

Prevention encompasses two basic ideas. First, that disease can be prevented by considering the physical, chemical, and emotional needs of the individual child. And second, that illness already begun can be prevented from progressing by using effective home care or professional care practices. In this chapter, prevention strategies falling into the first category will be discussed.

Breastfeeding

Breastfeeding is perhaps the most effective means of preventing not only middle ear infection, but infections of all types. Dr. R.K. Chandra, in three separate studies, investigated the effect of breastfeeding on the incidence of infection and allergy. He demonstrated, in India, that breastfed infants had a lower incidence of otitis media and respiratory infections (and diarrhea, dehydration, and pneumonia) than did children who were not breastfed. In Canada, breastfeeding was again associated with a decrease in the occurrence of otitis media and respiratory infection.[1, 2]

Dr. Chandra also showed that when newborn siblings of children with allergic disease are exclusively breastfed for a minimum of six weeks, the number of allergic indicators, including lowered antibodies to cow's milk, are significantly reduced.[3]

The duration of breastfeeding also appears to have an impact on the development of otitis media. Finnish researcher Dr. Ulla Saarinen followed 256 babies, born in the same three months, for one year. Of those breastfed for more than 6 months, only 6 percent had suffered an attack of otitis by the age of one year, in contrast to 19 percent of bottle-fed infants. Six percent of the children who had prolonged breastfeeding suffered four or more attacks of otitis media between one and three years of age, compared with 26 percent who had early introduction of cow's milk. Dr. Saarinen concluded that early and prolonged breastfeeding exerts a protective effect (against otitis media) that lasts up to three years.[4]

Dr. Michael Persico, in a study of 108 children with recurrent acute otitis media, found that 81 percent of the children who were not breastfed, or who were breastfed for less than three months, had their first episode of acute otitis media before the third month of life, in contrast to only 19 percent of children breastfed for more than three months.[5]

I encourage mothers to breastfeed for a minimum of six months. Breastfeeding for six to nine months is preferred. One year or more is ideal, but many mothers find it impractical. Concerns have been raised over the inability of human milk to supply adequate iron in children exclusively breastfed. However, the iron in breastmilk is sufficient to prevent anemia, for up to nine months. In addition, the mean hemoglobin concentration has been shown to be higher in breastfed infants than in iron-supplemented children at four and six months.

Whatever length of time you choose to breastfeed, keep in mind that lactation is very nutritionally demanding for a mother. To ensure that your baby continues to receive adequate amounts of zinc, iron, fatty acids and other nutrients, you must maintain a diet which is high in these nutrients. A multivitamin supplement (one that is free of sugar, wheat, dairy, yeast, additives, etc.) coupled with a balanced diet is an advisable way to replace the nutrients lost during lactation.

Avoid megavitamin supplementation or single nutrient supplementation during lactation. Not only do nutrients taken in excess go directly into the breastmilk, but some can even inhibit lactation. For example, mothers frequently need additional vitamin B6 during pregnancy and following delivery. However, if B6 is taken in excess (150-200 mg/day), it can inhibit lactation.

Because of the tendency for the breastmilk of American mothers to be deficient in fatty acids, I advise lactating mothers to take one tablespoon of flax oil and three capsules of primrose oil daily.

Occasionally, breastfed infants will develop recurrent otitis media. When this occurs, it is usually due to a food (or foods) in the mother's diet to which either the mother or the child is allergic. Challenge feeding tests can usually be used to identify sensitivities to foods. Once the offending food is identified, it can be eliminated from the diet. If challenge feeding (elimination-provocation) yields no clear results, your child may have a nutritional need that is not being met. This can sometimes be difficult to solve. In cases like this, make sure that fatty acid and zinc intake is sufficient. Finding a doctor knowledgeable in nutrition is important.

Feeding Position

Avoid feeding your baby a bottle while she is lying on her back in the crib, playpen, or anywhere else. Feeding in this position *increases* the likelihood that formula will reflux (or back up) into the eustachian tube. I advise mothers to treat their bottlefed baby as a nursing mother would treat her suckling infant. A nursing mother does not have the option of lying her child down (separately) while feeding. The mother and baby remain in close contact at all times. This provides not only a nourishing experience for the child, but a nurturing one for both mother and child. A mother who bottlefeeds her child should take the same opportunity to nurture by holding her child while feeding the bottle.

Preventing Airborne Allergy and Otitis Media

Reducing the level of airborne allergens in the home can be an important part of preventing recurrent earaches, especially (but not only) in children who have known airborne allergies. Here are some considerations:

Electrostatic Furnace Filter

These remove allergens and microbes from the air with electrically charged plates. The positively charged debris is attracted to the negatively charged plates, and the negatively charged debris is attracted to the positively charged plates. These can go a long way toward purifying the stale and polluted air in a home during winter. These filters have one major drawback—a fair amount of maintenance is required to keep the precipitators free of debris. But if they are well-maintained, electrostatic filters can reduce respiratory problems (including otitis) considerably.

These devices are also helpful in summer if central air conditioning is used. Electrostatic air cleaners are essential for children with known airborne allergies, but are recommended for any household since particulates in the winter or summer can irritate the mucous membranes of even healthy individuals.

Negative Ion Generator

These devices emit a stream of negatively charged ions that cause positively charged debris to precipitate out of the air (with the aid of a filter). Research I and my colleagues conducted with a Minnesota university showed negative ion generators coupled with filtration to be one of the most effective ways of removing bacteria, mold, fungi, and dust from the air. Negative ion generators are extremely efficient at removing cigarette smoke (although it is no substitute for the cessation of smoking).

Ion generators are practical in a room to room setting. They must be coupled with a filter (preferably an Electret™* filter) to provide any real benefit.

Woodstoves and Fireplaces

These should be well-built with a source of outside air. A University of Michigan study showed that the incidence of upper respiratory problems was significantly greater in children living where woodstoves were used in the home. Fireplace centers can assist homeowners in the specifics of attaching an outside air source to their woodstove or fireplace. This is essential in all homes, not only in those where children exhibit illness.

In 1985, one of my patients lamented that each of his three children was sick with something nearly all winter long. Two of the boys had chronic recurrent ear infections and the third suffered from bronchitis. After questioning the father for some time, it appeared that the woodstove they were using might be responsible for his children's ongoing health problems. I suggested that he disconnect the woodstove (which was their primary source of heat) and use their backup system for the next month. Within two weeks, all children showed improvement. By the fifth week, things were back to normal for the family except for an occasional cold. This family had a woodstove that was inefficient and poorly ventilated. The gases and particulates that had built up inside the home as a result of burning were a source of constant upper respiratory irritation to the children.

It is advisable to have a negative ion generator operating in the room where your fireplace or woodstove is burning. This

---

*The Electret filter is made by 3M. It consists of positively charged and negatively charged fibers interwoven in a tight pattern. The filters work by trapping debris as with normal filters. In addition, the charged fibers attract charged particles that stick to the fibers.

will help to filter most of the soot, smoke, and particulates that inevitably end up in the house because of burning.

Household Dampness

Damp areas should be eliminated and the sources identified. Mold and mildew are often imperceptible either by sight or smell, but can aggravate persistent middle ear problems in sensitive children. The bathroom, basement, and kitchen are the most likely areas.

Volatile Indoor Air Pollutants

In chapter 5, I described the manner in which volatile organic vapors can cause irritation of the upper respiratory tract and middle ear. The items that contribute to this should be identified and removed from the home. These include waxes, polishes, varnish, paint, cleaning solutions, old newsprint, and much more. The table listed in chapter 5 is a useful general guide to the substances containing volatile compounds.[6] For alternatives to some of the toxic products found in the home, I suggest you read *The Non-Toxic Home* and *Non-Toxic and Natural*, both by Debra Lynn Dadd.

Vacuum Cleaners and Carpeting

Dr. Edward Kenny, of the York Research Laboratory, claims that rugs and carpets test about 20 times dirtier than the average city sidewalk.[7] The carpet is where infants and toddlers spend most of their time, so ensuring a clean play area is crucial. Typical "bag filter" vacuum cleaners are notorious for moving more dust around the home than almost any other source. They are also a harbor for housemites, bacteria, and antigens. (See chapter 3.)

To solve this problem, many allergists recommend a "water vacuum" for cleaning homes. In a study by the Missouri State Medical Association, it was discovered that the Rainbow Vacuum (Rexair Corporation) can reduce the household dust concentration to one-fifth the amount that exists when ordinary bag-type vacuum cleaners are used. Another acceptable option is a central vacuum system with an outside exhaust.

Air-to-Air Heat Exchanger
These units function to bring fresh air into the home during the winter with only minimal heat loss. By continuously removing stale air and bringing in fresh, the number of air-borne irritants is reduced.

Air Travel

While not a significant contributor to otitis media, flying in an airplane can result in considerable distress for many children. Because of the rapid change in pressure, the eustachian tube sometimes does not open properly. To prevent problems with air travel, an infant should be nursed, given a pacifier, or given a bottle upon take-off and landing. Older children can be given a beverage to sip or gum to chew.

Smoking

The evidence linking smoking and childhood otitis media is indisputable. Cigarette smoke is among the most significant respiratory irritants found indoors. Its ability to cause otitis media in children is well documented. The solution for parents who smoke is to either quit smoking or smoke outside the home. If you choose to continue smoking in the presence of your child, first consider the adverse effects of smoking on the ears and then the added adverse effects of repeated antibiotics (to which your child will likely be subjected). Also consider that the alternative methods described in this book may be significantly *less* effective if you continue to smoke.

The Day Care Dilemma

The number of children spending time in day care grows each year. Health officials estimate that by the year 1995, two-thirds of all preschool children and three-quarters of all school age children will need some sort of child care while their parents work.[8] With this rise in day care usage comes an increased risk of illness to the children who participate.

Infants and toddlers in day care settings are twice as likely as those in home care to contract an illness that lasts more than 10 days, causes a fever of at least 102 degrees for three or more days, or requires medical attention.[9] For a variety of reasons, germs easily spread from child to child in the close quarters of the day care setting. A variety of infectious organisms have been isolated from day care workers and children. Among the most common are:[10]

- *Giardia lamblia*
- *Shigella*
- *Salmonella*
- *Escherichia coli*
- *Entamoeba histolytica*
- *Adenoviruses*
- *Rotavirus*
- *Haemophilus influenzae*
- *Streptococcus pneumoniae*

Dr. Stanley Schuman, of the Medical University of South Carolina, blames day care centers for "outbreaks of illness—diarrhea, dysentery, giardiasis, and epidemic jaundice—reminiscent of the pre-sanitation days of the 17th century."[11] A study published in 1984 revealed that children in day care centers were more than 12 times as likely to be infected with *Hemophilus influenzae* type b.[12] Another showed that day care children are 15 to 20 times more likely to contract giardiasis than children under maternal home care.[13]

Researchers at the University of Alabama found that 59 percent of day care children were shedding cytomegalovirus.

Cytomegalovirus (CMV) was found on toys and other items frequently handled by children in the day care center. Based on antibody testing, it was estimated that between 70 and 100 percent of day care children were infected with CMV.[14]

A study reported in the *American Journal of Public Health* in 1988 compared children raised at home, raised in another home, and placed in nursery school or day care. The investigators in this study found that, compared to children reared at home, children in day care spent 30 percent more sick days in bed, while those raised in another home spent 19 percent more sick days in bed. Children in day care were also likely to spend more time in hospitals than children raised at home.[15, 16]

A number of studies have shown that otitis media occurs more frequently in day care children than in children minded at home.[17, 18] Drs. L. Birch and O. Elbrond compared the rate of otitis media in children minded exclusively at home with those spending time in day care. They found the occurrence of otitis media to be significantly higher in those attending day care centers. Moreover, long-lasting episodes of otitis media were found to be considerably more common among the children in day care centers.[19] A 1988 report in the *Journal of Pediatrics* revealed that hospitalization for myringotomy and tube placement occurred in 21 percent of the children in day care compared with only 3 percent of those in home care.[20]

Day care is here to stay. Many families require two incomes in order to survive. Certainly, many single parents would find it impossible to work or go to school without available day care for their children. Even the federal government has expressed its need to have mothers in the work force. However, the health implications of the growing day care situation are enormous. Public health officials are working to stem the rising tide of infections in day care children. At this stage there seems to be little progress. Some have recommended mass immunization of day care children, but this carries with it a host of social, philosophical, and medical implications.

Parents and day care providers should be aware of things

they can do to reduce the spread of infectious disease. For parents, it is necessary to be aware of times when your child should be kept out of day care. For providers, it is important to know which children should be excluded or sent home. These are only first steps since the nature of the day care environment contributes to the spread of illness among children.

Recognize that otitis media is not considered a communicable disease in the strict sense. Yet, many of the conditions that predispose children to the development of middle ear effusion are considered communicable. The following guidelines are useful in determining when to exclude children from day care. For more information, contact your local community health department.

Guidelines For Excluding From Day Care
Children who have the following symptoms should be excluded from the child care setting until 1) a physician has certified the symptoms are not associated with an infectious agent or the child is no longer a threat to the health of other children at the center, or 2) the symptoms have subsided.

For the mildly ill child, exclusion should be based on whether there are adequate facilities and staff available to meet the needs of both the ill child and other children in the group.

FEVER   *Axillary* or *oral* temperature: 100 degrees F. or higher, or *Rectal* temperature: 101 degrees F. or higher; especially if accompanied by other symptoms such as vomiting, sore throat, diarrhea, headache and stiff neck, or undiagnosed rash.

RESPIRATORY SYMPTOMS   Difficult or rapid breathing or severe coughing:
— child makes high-pitched croupy or whooping sound after he coughs.

	—child unable to lie comfortably due to continuous cough.
DIARRHEA	An increased number of abnormally loose stools in the previous 24 hours. Observe the child for other symptoms such as fever, abdominal pain, or vomiting.
VOMITING	Two or more episodes of vomiting within the previous 24 hours.
EYE/NOSE DRAINAGE	Thick mucus or pus draining from the eye or nose.
SORE THROAT	Sore throat, especially when fever or swollen glands in the neck are present.
SKIN PROBLEMS	Rash—Skin rashes, undiagnosed or contagious. Infected sores—Sores with crusty, yellow or green drainage which cannot be covered by clothing or bandages.
ITCHING	Persistent itching (or scratching) of body or scalp.
APPEARANCE, BEHAVIOR	Child looks or acts differently: unusually tired, pale, lacking appetite. Confused, irritable, difficult to awaken.
UNUSUAL COLOR	Eyes or skin—yellow (jaundice) Stool—Gray or white Urine—Dark, tea-colored These symptoms can be found in hepatitis and should be evaluated by a physician.

Reprinted with permission from "*Infectious Diseases in Child-care Settings: Information for Directors, Caregivers, and Parents or Guardians,*" prepared by the Epidemiology Departments of: Hennepin County Community Health, St. Paul Division of Public Health, Minnesota Department of Health, Washington County Public Health, Bloomington Division of Health. These guidelines are not to be considered all-inclusive. They are subject to ongoing revision as more information becomes available.

The Day Care Diet
Be aware of what your child is being fed while attending day care. Cheese, cold apple juice, and peanut butter sandwiches are common fare. However, consumption of these foods on a daily basis can irritate a toddler's digestive system and be a contributor to recurring illness. Determine the foods that best suit your child's specific needs and make arrangements to have this incorporated in to your child's daily routine. Give your day care provider a list of foods that you wish your child to avoid. This may include foods to which your child is allergic or those that are not optimal for a child's digestion.

Dietary Considerations

Changing and improving dietary habits can be an important step in the prevention of recurrent earaches.

Early Introduction of Solid Foods
Solids should not be introduced before your child is six months of age (see *shi fan* below). Earlier introduction solid food often contributes to health problems, including the development of allergies and earaches.

Introduction of Solid Foods
When beginning to introduce solid foods into a baby's diet, it is important that only one food at a time be added. This way, if your child is sensitive to that food, you can identify it and

avoid feeding it. Once your child's digestive tract has matured somewhat, you may wish to introduce the food again. Introduce the least allergenic foods first. The first solids your baby eats should *not* be from among the most common offenders. These include:

- Dairy products.
- Wheat.
- Eggs.
- Chocolate.
- Citrus.
- Corn.
- Soy.
- Peanuts and other nuts.
- Shellfish.
- Sugar.
- Yeast.

Fruit Juice

Most children consume far too much fruit juice. A glass of juice is almost purely simple carbohydrate—in other words, sugar. Excess sugar leads to deficiencies in immune function, as described above. If you must give fruit juice, dilute it 1:1 with water, and don't give it cold out of the refrigerator. Most parents go to great lengths to make sure their baby's formula is warm, but think nothing of feeding a bottle of cold juice from the refrigerator. Cold juice can slow digestion in a child of any age.

Honey

Often, parents feel they are doing their child a service by feeding honey instead of sugar. This is a mistake if large quantities of honey are given, since honey contains the same sugar found in table sugar. There is an interesting phenomenon surrounding honey. When beekeepers want to calm the hive, they mix a solution of sugar water and spray the bees. A solution of water and *raw* honey also has a calming effect on the bees. However, when pasteurized honey is used, all bees exposed will be found dead within 20 minutes.[21] It is unclear why this occurs, but it seems to suggest that raw honey may be a better dietary choice for humans than pasteurized honey. Almost all honey you find in the grocery stores is pasteurized. You have to look specifically for raw honey. A good place to start is a local food co-op or health food store.

Treat honey as you would any sugar and use it sparingly, especially if your child is ill. *Recognize that most doctors advise against feeding honey to children under one year.*

Sugar

I treat this separately because sugar is added to nearly every type of packaged food available in stores. A study by Cheraskin and Ringsdorf has shown that when sugar is ingested, the ability of white blood cells to destroy bacteria can fall by as much as 60 percent.[22] Excessive sugar inhibits fatty acid metabolism (discussed in chapter 5) because it is high in calories but lacks the nutrients needed to make the enzymes work properly. High intake of sugar also increases the need for magnesium and increases the amount of magnesium excreted in the urine.[23, 24]

I suggest you read labels carefully. Any time sugar appears among the top five or six ingredients, don't buy the product.

Variety of Foods

Avoid feeding the same foods every day. Food sensitivity can be induced by overconsuming a given food every day for a long period. The solution is to rotate foods. Instead of feeding oatmeal every morning for breakfast, feed oatmeal one day, wheat cereal the next, fruit the next, and so on. With infants, rice is preferable to wheat.

If your child has known food allergies, don't feed those foods more than once or twice a week. When you do feed them, give only small amounts.

Cooked Food

Avoid feeding raw food to your infant. Fruits need not be cooked, but vegetables and other foods should be. Raw foods are more difficult to digest. They're also more apt to contribute to allergy. Also, cold food should not be fed to a child. When food is eaten cold the body must first warm it to almost 100 degrees (F) before it can be properly utilized. For an infant or child whose digestive system is immature, this can spell trouble.

Infant Formula

If you choose not to breastfeed, you should know a few things about infant formula. Powdered formula mix is higher in oxidized fats than is liquid formula. As I stated in chapter 5, oxidized fats in the diet can set the stage for inflammation and immune function problems. Some infant formulas contain aluminum in concentrations 30 to 100 times greater than that found in human milk. Aluminum is a toxic metalloid that has been implicated in brain and kidney damage.[25, 26] For healthy infants this may not be a serious problem since the blood levels of aluminum following ingestion of formula are no higher than that of breastfed infants. At this time the issue is not clear.[27]

The greatest drawback of infant formula (following the absence of immune components) is the significant lack of the proper fatty acids. Most formula is too low in omega-3 and omega-6 fatty acids. Soy formulas are undesirable because of their low carnitine content. Additionally, several days after the processing of soybeans into milk, toxic metabolites develop that can impair digestion.

Cow's milk causes allergic reactions in a large percentage of children. Cow's milk and most milk-based formulas (except Enfamil) contain insufficient amounts of the amino acid taurine. Taurine deficiency has been linked to the development of inflammatory conditions, which may be one reason cow's milk consumption gives rise to increased rates of infection and inflammation. If you choose to feed your child cow's milk, use whole milk rather than skim or low-fat milk (1% or 2%). Low-fat milk has a high protein-to-fat ratio which is not suitable for children. Consumption of low-fat milk by children can cause kidney stress.

Dr. Leo Galland, a respected pediatrician and nutrition researcher, recommends the use of milk-based formula over soy-based formula. Of the most popular brands, he suggests using Similac as a first choice. If your child cannot digest it, switch to Enfamil.[28]

In China, mothers commonly feed their babies *shi fan*, or rice soup, either as the child's first solid food or as a substitute for formula. It is made by cooking one part *brown* rice to six parts water at low temperature for several hours or overnight. Cooking for a lengthy period causes the rice to break down into a thin, milky soup not unlike breastmilk in consistency. The soup is well-tolerated by most children and helps to prepare the child's immature digestive tract for digestion of solid foods. As the child ages she can be given soup which has been thickened by adding less water. Eventually, cooked vegetables such as carrots can be added to the soup.[29]

Essential Fatty Acids

As I mentioned in chapter 5, the amount of important omega-3 fatty acids in our diet has declined by 80 percent over the past 100 years. Omega-6 fatty acid consumption has remained relatively constant during this time, but because of other factors these fatty acids are not properly converted into prostaglandins. Therefore, a good prevention program consists of adding a small amount of omega-3 oils to your child's diet each day (especially if he has a history of allergies, skin problems, or infections).

The best vegetable source of omega-3 fatty acids is flax oil (not commercial linseed oil). I recommend the oil made by Spectrum Natural. (See resources.) It can be given 1 teaspoon twice a day.

Another option is to give fish oil, which is high in EPA.

Most fish oil comes in large capsules. Rather than attempting to get your child to swallow a capsule (which is dangerous for any child under five), I suggest you break the capsule open and mix it in juice. EPA will taste fishy, so it may be objectionable to many children.

Cod liver oil is another good source of omega-3 fatty acids. It is also high in vitamin A and D. The main problem is that if you give too much cod liver oil for too long, the levels of A and D can become toxic. Giving 1 teaspoon of cod liver oil every three or four days is a safe level for most children.

As discussed in chapter 5, the enzyme necessary for proper conversion of fatty acids is inactive in infants and is frequently blocked in older children. So it may be helpful to give periodic doses of gamma-linolenic acid (GLA). Evening primrose oil is the best source of GLA. Borage oil is another good source. One perle can be given every other day in a prevention program. It is best to open the perle and give the oil rather than having your small child try to swallow it. Any formula-fed baby may need to be given GLA if he has health problems.

Never use the essential fatty acids I've discussed for cooking. They break down quickly when exposed to heat. They also break down when exposed to air. They should be stored in a brown bottle and refrigerated always. When taken out of the refrigerator, the amount needed should be taken and the cover quickly replaced. Some suggest breaking open a capsule of vitamin E and placing the contents into your bottle of oil for better storage.

Always give additional vitamin E (25 I.U./day) when you feed your child essential fatty acids.

Trans Fatty Acids

Avoid feeding your child any of the non-essential fatty acids or foods containing partially hydrogenated oils. Foods to be avoided include:

- Cookies, pastries, doughnuts.
- Candy bars.
- Some crackers.
- French fries, potato cakes, chicken nuggets.
- Deep-fried fish sandwiches.
- Margarine.
- Vegetable shortening.
- Corn chips, potato chips.
- Cake frostings.
- Malt balls (carob or chocolate).

Read labels! If the label says "may contain the following," be suspicious. If the "following" includes the words *partially hydrogenated*, avoid the product. Cottonseed oil, palm kernel oil, and coconut oil are also used frequently in packaged foods. Avoid these as well, since they are saturated fats that may interfere with the enzyme delta-6-desaturase, needed to convert fatty acids into prostaglandins.

It might seem that eliminating these foods from the diet would take some fun out of life. Indeed, the list includes many childhood favorites. However, recurrent illness is no fun either. Any substantial reduction in the non-essential fats will go a long way toward improving your child's resistance to disease.

Drinking Water

Do not allow your child to drink soft water. Soft water contributes to magnesium loss and may contain excess sodium and aluminum. The most desirable alternatives are distilled water and water purified using a combination of carbon filtration and reverse osmosis.

Tap water often contains high levels of chlorine (for antibacterial purposes). The chlorine in tap water is believed by some to inhibit the beneficial bacteria in the intestines. In addition, when chlorine combines with organic matter present in water, it is converted to chloroform—a highly toxic substance.

Lead is another toxic element commonly found in tap water. Lead leaches into the water from pipe joints that have been soldered using leaded materials (which is common). Since you cannot be sure if your water contains lead without having it tested, I recommend that you let the water run for three or four minutes every morning before using it. This will purge most of the lead from the water that has been standing overnight. Anytime your water has not been used for six or eight hours (or more), the water should be purged in this way.

Reduce Your Child's Intake of Canned Food

The average daily intake of tin (from canned food) is 200 mg/day.[30] Tin is a known inhibitor of zinc and selenium, both of which play important roles in immune function and prevention of inflammation. In addition, canned foods contain considerable amounts of lead (used as solder), which has immune-inhibiting effects. The amount of lead found in canned tuna, for instance, is 10,000 times the amount of lead found in fresh tuna.[31] Complete avoidance is not practical or necessary, but I would restrict the intake of canned foods.

Avoid Soft Drinks

I'm constantly amazed at the amount of soft drinks parents give to young children. The average soft drink contains 9 teaspoons of sugar. In addition, some (especially cola) contain high amounts of phosphoric acid, which binds with magnesium and pulls it out of the body. One 12-ounce can of cola contains 36 mg of phosphoric acid, which displaces 36 mg of magnesium. (Non-cola beverages often use ascorbic acid instead of phosphoric acid. Ascorbic acid does not have the same effect.) The importance of magnesium in fatty acid metabolism is described in chapter 5.

Intestinal Bacteria

Children who are formula-fed are usually deficient in the bacteria *L. acidophilus* and *B. bifidus*. In breastfed babies, the numbers of these bacteria are high, but fall off once breastfeeding is stopped. Any child who has been on antibiotics probably needs *bifidobacteria*. Children in whom formula was introduced early in life also require *bifidus*. One teaspoon per day is an acceptable prevention dose.

Vitamins and Minerals

If your child consumes a diet consisting of whole foods, the need for additional vitamins and minerals should be minimal. A multivitamin supplement is usually all that is necessary unless there are obvious signs of nutritional deficiency. Be aware that many of the popular children's vitamins are loaded with sugar. I think this is unacceptable. When you choose a children's vitamin, read the label and be sure it contains no added sugar. Also be certain it contains no soy, yeast, wheat, milk, dyes, or other additives. This is especially important in a child with allergies.

What to Feed Your Child

Although this section contains "wisdom" about dietary practices that will help prevent ear infections, it is probably the Chinese to whom we should look for advice on proper eating. Acupuncturist Bob Flaws wrote in the *American Journal of Acupuncture* in 1989, "While interning at the Yue Yang Hospital with Dr. Chen [Li-chen] in 1984, I did not see a single case of pediatric otitis media." While gathered with senior physicians at the hospital, Flaws was asked what was the most common pediatric problem in the United States. His response was "earache." The Chinese pediatric specialists agreed that earaches were not much of a problem in China.[32]

These doctors attribute the low rate of otitis media in Chinese children to the way food is cooked, combined, and introduced into their children's diets. In contrast, Chinese doctors studying in the West conclude that our children are being fed in a way that promotes the development of illness. I have to agree!

Chinese medicine has evolved through centuries of practice and observation. The dietary practices of the Chinese people have emerged from the same philosophical framework. As a student and practitioner of both Chinese and Western medicine I have learned that these time-honored traditions have an inherent wisdom and stability that in many ways surpasses our own. In my opinion, following the general principles of Chinese dietary practices can have a substantial impact on the health of children in the West.

It is beyond the scope of this book to discuss the details of food preparation and combining. For more information on Chinese dietary practices I suggest you read *Prince Wen Hui's Cook: Chinese Dietary Therapy* by Bob Flaws. For a Western perspective on diet and nutrition that includes food lists, menus, and other valuable dietary recommendations, I suggest you read *Superimmunity for Kids* by Leo Galland, M.D., and *The Omega-3 Phenomenon* by Donald O. Rudin, M.D.

Minor Injuries

In chapter 5, I described how biomechanical problems can lead to the development of middle ear problems in your child. Biomechanical problems can be identified and corrected at any time following an injury, but are best corrected soon after the injury occurs and before ear problems arise.

Following Birth
Following the birth of your child is the optimum time to have him examined for biomechanical problems of the spine.

An examination for biomechanical problems of the spine is essential:

- If the birth has been particularly long and difficult.

- If forceps or vacuum extraction have been used to assist delivery.

- If there are sensory or motor problems of the head and neck.

- In cases of infantile torticollis (where the child's head appears to be fixed in or favoring one direction).

- Where chronic infections of the upper respiratory tract exist from birth (including chronic stuffiness or sinus congestion).

Examination of the spine is advised:

- After every birth. Even the normal forces of uterine contraction can disrupt the delicate spinal biomechanics of a newborn.

Following Injury

Any slip or fall has the potential to cause disruption in the normal function of the spinal biomechanics. Those which are more serious are obviously also the ones that have a greater likelihood of contributing to problems. Even minor falls can disrupt the spinal mechanics enough to affect the middle ear and surrounding tissues.

Examination is essential:

- When your child has taken a serious fall such as down the stairs, on the ice, off the changing table, or off the couch.

- If your child complains of headache or neck stiffness following a fall (especially if the complaints last for more than a few days).

- If your child complains of ringing in the ears or dizziness following a fall.

Examination is recommended:

- Whenever you sense that something is not quite right following a fall. If you notice behavior changes, change in posture, change in eating habits, change in hearing, etc., you should consider having your child examined.

An examination for biomechanical problems of the spine is typically done by a doctor of chiropractic or doctor of osteopathy. (Both are licensed to practice in all 50 states.) Don't be surprised if you take your child into your family medical doctor and he declares your child to be free of any problems following a fall. He is trained to look for pathology. He will check reflexes, check for fractures, check for concussion, and for any other signs that would suggest serious damage. Your medical doctor is not looking for functional changes in the mechanics of the spinal column. The chiropractor or osteopath, while also checking for signs of more serious injury, will examine for changes in spinal biomechanics.

Treating Colds and Nasal Congestion

Roughly one-half of all middle ear problems are preceded by colds, nasal congestion, or another upper respiratory problem. Thus, an important preventive measure is to treat these conditions quickly before they begin to involve the middle ear. Because most of these conditions are viral in origin, allopathic medicine lacks an effective therapy. This is where homeopathic medicine is often at its best.

When your child develops a cold, it will be helpful to consider the other preventive measures described in this chapter. In the homeopathic care of cold, there are several remedies you will need to consider.

Homeopathic Single Remedies
Aconite

Used in the first 24 hours of a cold that is due to exposure to cold or wind. Often associated with high fever. Thirst and restlessness are usually present. A hoarse, dry, croupy cough that comes on suddenly may be present. A child will often experience fear, anxiety, and worry. They do not want to be touched. The mucous membranes are dry and the nose is stopped up. If there is nasal discharge, it is slight and watery. Occasionally, nasal discharge is bloody. Earache may be present.

Symptoms are worse: from dry, cold winds, tobacco smoke, in a warm room, and in evening and night.

Symptoms are better: in open air.

Allium cepa

Indicated when there is much sneezing associated with watery eyes and a runny nose. The nasal discharge tends to be clear, watery, and offensive. It is irritating to the upper lip and increases when entering a warm room. The eyes frequently burn from the profuse tearing. However, the tears do not irritate the skin around the eyes. Earache and shooting pains in the eustachian tube may occur. *Allium cepa* is commonly associated with hoarseness and a tickling sensation in the throat. This remedy is often used to treat the symptoms of hay fever.

Symptoms are worse: in warm room, toward evening.

Symptoms are better: in a cold room and open air.

Antimonium tartaricum

A useful remedy for coughs that come on gradually and are associated with rattling of mucus with little expectoration. These children are drowsy and weak. The face is cold, blue, and pale. There is often quivering of the chin and trembling throughout the body. *Antimonium tart* is used in the latter stages of respiratory problems that do not improve. These children often require medical attention.

Symptoms are worse: from warmth, lying down at night, damp cold weather, and in evening.

Symptoms are better: from expectoration and sitting up.

Arsenicum album

There is a profuse, watery nasal discharge with sore, burning nostrils. The nose feels stopped up. The eyes, which may be swollen, burn from offensive tears. This is a useful remedy for different types of coughs. There is burning in the chest. The cough may be worse after midnight or while lying on the back. Respiration is often accompanied by wheezing. Exhaustion, restlessness, and symptoms that are aggravated at night are important signs that *Arsenicum* is needed. These children are anxious and fearful. High fever is common.

Symptoms are worse: in a cold room, from cold or wet weather, and after cold food or drink.

Symptoms are better: from heat, warm drinks, and elevating the head.

Belladonna

This remedy is used in the early stages of a cold. The illness usually comes on rapidly with little warning. It is usually associated with hot, red skin, flushed face, glaring eyes, restless sleep, and hypersensitivity of all senses. The throat is hot and dry with swollen tonsils. Earache is common with *Belladonna*. There is hoarseness and dryness of the mucous membranes of the nose, throat, and trachea. There is usually fever present, but the skin is dry. There is commonly no thirst. The emotional symptoms are important with *Belladonna*. The child is almost unaware of what is going on around her. The acuteness of her senses may cause her to be agitated and furious, which may lead to outbursts of hitting or biting. These children may have fears of imaginary things, hallucinations, and delirium. The pupils are dilated.

Symptoms are worse: from touch, noise, draft, light,

odors, and lying down.

Symptoms are better: by sitting semi-erect.

Euphrasia

Symptoms are almost the reverse of *Allium cepa*. The nasal discharge is non-irritating. The eyes, which seem to water constantly, produce tears that are highly irritating. There may be a mild cough.

Symptoms are worse: in evening, indoors, in a warm room (although the nasal symptoms are made worse in open air, in the morning and from lying down).

Ferrum phosphoricum

Ferrum phosphoricum is used both for colds and otitis media. This remedy is indicated in the early stages of a cold. It is commonly used in anemic children (although this is not a prerequisite) or after *Belladonna* has failed to give relief. There is tickling in the chest accompanied by a hard, croupy cough.

Symptoms are worse: at night and from touch.

Symptoms are better: with cold applications.

Gelsemium

There is an irritating watery nasal discharge. The hallmark of this remedy is chills running up and down the spine. Pervading the child is a general sense of sluggishness, heaviness, and muscular weakness. The cold comes on gradually. Breathing is slow and labored.

Symptoms are worse: in damp weather.

Symptoms are better: in open air and with motion.

Hepar sulphuricum

This is also an important remedy for otitis media. It is used in the latter stages of a cold when the nasal discharge has become thick, yellowish, and offensive. These children are easily irritated and are hypersensitive to touch. The voice may be lost when exposed to dry, cold air. The cough is loose, rattling, and commonly worse in the morning. This child is so sensitive to cold that a hand or foot exposed from beneath the covers causes aggravation of the cough.

Symptoms are worse: from dry cold winds, cold foods, or the slightest draft.

Symptoms are better: from warmth, humidity, and after eating.

Kali bichromicum

Kali bic is not a typical cold remedy but is an extremely valuable remedy for sinus congestion. Pain is around the root of the nose. Nasal discharge is thick, ropy, and greenish-yellow. Violent sneezing is common.

Symptoms are worse: with cold (air and drink).

Symptoms are better: with warmth and pressure.

Natrum muriaticum

The child awakens with much sneezing. Heavy nasal discharge, described as having a raw egg-white appearance, is present. Small eruptions or vesicles form around the lips. The lips and corners of the mouth are dry, ulcerated, and cracked. A crack in the middle of the lower lip is sometimes seen. These children are irritable, weepy, and wish to be alone. Their symptoms may be aggravated when one attempts to console them.

Symptoms are worse: from noise, consolation, lying down, heat, talking, and in a warm room.

Symptoms are better: from cold bathing, lying on right side, going without regular meals, and in open air.

Nux vomica

This remedy is used after exposure to dry, cold weather. However, the symptoms do not come on as rapidly as with *Aconite*. Heavy nasal discharge is fluid during the daytime, but stuffed up at night. Discharge may alternate from left to right nostril. There is hoarseness with a sensation of scraping in the throat.

Nux children are irritable, sensitive and do not like to be touched. They are sensitive to noises, odors, and light. When a cough is present, it is worse after eating or upon waking. The cough is often dry and hacking. These children are greatly sensitive to cold.

Symptoms are worse: from touch, dry weather, cold, after eating, after mental work, and in the morning.

Symptoms are better: in the evening, while at rest, and after warm drinks.

Pulsatilla

This medicine is useful in acute otitis media but is also valuable for colds. There is thick, bland, yellowish-green discharge, sometimes accompanied by a dry or loose cough. There tends to be a dry cough in the evening and at night. In the morning there is a loose cough with copious expectoration of mucus. The nose is often stuffed at night. The child is weepy, easily discouraged, and melancholy. He is frequently feverish, but also thirstless. Symptoms improve markedly when he is outdoors. This child likes the head held high and often desires to sleep with more than one pillow.

Symptoms are worse: from heat, lying down, exertion, after eating, toward evening, and in a warm room.

Symptoms are better: with motion, cold applications, cold food and drink, and in open air.

Rhus toxicodendron

The nasal discharge is thick and yellow-green. The nose feels congested. A tickling sensation behind the breastbone is often accompanied by a dry, teasing cough from midnight until morning. *Rhus tox* is indicated for children who feel better when moving about. The remedy is often needed when there is itchiness of the skin.

Symptoms are worse: from cold, wet, rainy weather; during sleep, when lying on back, and at night.

Symptoms are better: from warm, dry weather; motion, walking, change of position, and warm applications.

Spongia

This is an important remedy for coughs that are dry, barking, and croupy. The cough usually improves after eating or drinking, especially warm drinks. There may be profuse nasal discharge alternating with blockage. These children are anxious and fearful. Any form of excitement aggravates their cough. They may awaken in the middle of the night with a fearful suffocating sensation.

Symptoms are worse: from wind, lying down, excitement, and before midnight.

Whenever a cough or cold becomes severe or is associated with vomiting, shortness of breath, or difficulty breathing, your physician should be consulted.

Down Syndrome

I am uncertain of the extent to which earaches can be prevented in children with Down syndrome or cleft palate since much of the problem is due to the structural configuration of the palate. However, there is evidence that children with Down syndrome may have nutritional requirements that are considerably different from other children. For this reason, you may want to consult a doctor knowledgeable in nutrition. Also, homeopathic constitutional care may provide some benefit.

Season

Earaches are less likely to occur during the summer months than at any other time during the year (although some children experience earaches year round). Throughout the year, it will be important to follow the dietary, feeding, and nutritional guidelines for prevention of earaches. As fall approaches (especially in temperate regions), taking the preventive steps regarding indoor air quality, indoor humidity, etc., will become important.

*   *   *

It is not possible to prevent the development of illness entirely. This is especially true in children because they are new creatures of this world. Every encounter with a strange bacterium or virus must by design arouse the defenses. This frequently manifests in symptoms that appear for a short time and then disappear, the battle having been won. This process is an essential part of developing the immune recognition system. This type of illness is expected. The illness we hope to prevent is that which is recurrent or that which lingers, gradually taking the strength from the sick child.

Chapter 8

Alternative Treatment: Some Solutions

*"There is no longer any doubt about the value of incor-
porating traditional medicine into modern health care."* [1]
Olayiwola Akerele, World Health Organization

Childhood otitis media is often as frustrating for doctors to treat
as it is for parents to endure. There are those within medicine
who are confident that the current state of treatment is effective
and safe. Moreover, the public generally believes that there is
a consensus among doctors regarding the safety, efficacy, and
application of these methods. A look at the evidence presented
in chapters 2 and 3 suggests, however, that there are many
voices of dissension regarding the treatment of otitis media.
Recall the following remarks by respected investigators in the
fields of pediatrics and otolaryngology:

"The treatment of recurrent otitis media remains an unresolved
problem." [2]

"There is no consensus of opinion regarding effective medical
treatment of secretory otitis media." [3]

". . . secretory otitis media is a self-limiting disease, which is
not affected by any of the current methods of treatment." [4]

"Otitis media with effusion . . . appears to be more common
since the widespread use of antibiotics." [5]

What do these statements imply about the current state of treatment of otitis media? At the very least, they suggest that there is room for improvement—a niche which holistic methods might arguably fill. At best, comments such as these should cause us to consider fundamental changes in the clinical management of otitis media. It may be time to step back and reassess the problem. It may be time to embrace the holistic viewpoint. It may indeed be time to take a serious look at the holistic models already in place and determine what role they may play in the effective management of a problem in urgent need of solutions.

In this chapter are presented the most common and most effective methods used in the holistic management of otitis media. Based on anecdotal evidence and clinical case studies, the methods described below have been shown to have significant value in the care of otitis media. Admittedly, there is not sufficient scientific research on these methods at present. It is my hope that this chapter will serve as the foundation upon which further investigation into alternatives is based.

Using This Chapter

This section is intended primarily for health practitioners who want access to a resource for the care of otitis media. While this section is written for clinicians, there is a wealth of information useful to parents. Without a clinical background, however, it may be difficult to make practical use of the information.

In providing this information, I assume that:

- Anyone using this information has formal training in the health sciences.

- Anyone attempting to manage otitis media conduct an otoscopic examination (and a complete physical exam) on each child before engaging in any form of treatment. And that such persons be aware of the diagnostic implications of the various findings on otoscopic examination.

- Anyone using this information has training in one or more of the specialties described below.

- Anyone managing otitis media be fully aware of the potential for complications and the signs and symptoms associated with those complications.

Alternative Treatment Methods Described

The methods of management described below have been established based on clinical observation. They have been compiled from a variety of sources. To my knowledge, they have not been subjected to double-blind, placebo-controlled study in otitis media. Descriptions of each form of therapy are provided to show the detailed approaches used to treat otitis media and to serve as a background for those wishing to know more about specific diagnosis and treatment.

Information in this chapter is presented for educational purposes only. It is not to be construed as recommendation for treatment and is not intended to replace the clinical judgment of the physician. No claims of the ability to cure otitis media are made. Moreover, the information contained in this chapter should not be viewed as all-inclusive. Although I have attempted to provide a wide survey of the alternative methods used to manage otitis media, there may be others I have omitted.

The benefit of the methods described below is that they can be used to successfully treat constitutional weaknesses that typically predispose children to the development of otitis media. A profound example of recovery using holistic methods was reported to me by Dr. Martha Benedict. She describes the case of a two-year-old boy with recurrent otitis media. The boy had been on repeated antibiotics for some time. His infections had persisted for so long that the eardrum had almost completely dissolved. A look into the ear canal revealed virtually no eardrum. The ear ossicles were directly visible. The child's otolaryngologist began talk of surgically implanting a prosthetic eardrum.

Dr. Benedict began her treatment, which consisted of botanical medicine and dietary management. She described the child's diet as full of sugar and white flour. After several months of treatment, the earaches began to subside. What's most remarkable about this case is that Dr. Benedict observed a gradual regeneration of the eardrum. Over time, the eardrum was almost completely restored by natural means. I share this story not to imply that eardrums can be regenerated by diet and herbs, but to illustrate the remarkable healing ability of the body once constitutional weaknesses are overcome.

Listed below are six forms of alternative treatment currently used to manage otitis media. The philosophical and scientific basis behind each method of treatment is thoroughly described elsewhere and will not be presented here.

The six methods are:

- Allergy Management.
- Homeopathic Medicine.
- Manipulation.
- Acupuncture.
- Botanical Medicine.
- Clinical Nutrition.

Allergy Management

The clinical management of allergy is complex. To address it in sufficient depth would require another book the size of this one. It would, therefore, be presumptuous of me to attempt a detailed discussion of clinical allergy management. I have chosen instead to comment on the importance of addressing constitutional weaknesses in the child and outline the forms of allergy tests currently available.

The Constitutional Approach

Constitution refers to the child's (or any person's) general level of health. It takes into consideration his lifestyle, environmental influences, history of past illness, heredity, and even parental history of illness. Constitutional treatment is directed toward the management of these areas and toward restoring vigor to the body systems that are weak, damaged, or poorly functioning. Constitutional treatment is, therefore, not considered acute care. The use of constitutional treatment can take place alongside acute care.

Constitutional care also might be viewed as any effort to correct underlying metabolic problems. In this section, I will briefly address some underlying metabolic considerations in approaching the management of both airborne allergy (or hypersensitivity) and food allergy (or hypersensitivity). This is not intended to be a practical discussion, but more of a survey.

Indoor Air Pollution and Hypersensitivity

Vapors from chemicals such as benzene, toluene, and formaldehyde are found with increasing regularity in the air inside our homes. These compounds can cause mucous membrane inflammation in the eyes, ears, nose, throat, and lungs of most individuals exposed. In individuals sensitive to these compounds, severe hypersensitivity or allergic reactions can occur with exposure to only tiny amounts of such vapors. This includes adverse reactions of the immune system.

To deal with these compounds, the body has several separate defensive systems in place. One is the mixed function oxidase system (MFO), and another is the antioxidant defense system. When exposed to airborne pollutants, these systems go to work converting the chemicals into usually harmless substances that can be eliminated from the body. Some chemicals are converted into substances more toxic than those originally inhaled. Many compounds act as free radicals (discussed in chapter 5). The demands placed on the defensive system are considerable, but not overwhelming.

When exposure to such substances occurs over time—which happens in cases of urban air pollution or indoor air pollution—the defensive systems are overwhelmed and the antioxidants are depleted. What the body must do is shift, or shunt, its defensive platoons to those areas of the body that are receiving the greatest exposure. In our example, this is the lungs since the substances are breathed. By shifting defenses to the lungs, the body, in essence, reduces its defenses in other areas.[6]

The problem is that we are being exposed to similar substances through the food and water. This is especially true when diets are high in oxidized fats, or trans fatty acids. When diets are deficient in the raw materials—nutrients—needed to make the defensive systems work, the damaging effects of exposure to toxic substances are amplified.

What this means is that there may be an ever-increasing number of children sensitive to a wide variety of substances in their environment. Continued low-level exposure to toxic substances coupled with inadequate dietary intake of the vitamins and minerals needed to metabolize these substances may lead to increased reactivity to the environment (food, pollens, chemicals, etc.), greater immune compromise, susceptibility to infection, and susceptibility to inflammation.

Food Allergy

Many doctors argue that the incidence of food allergy is rising rapidly. Some contend that the rise is due to the increasing use of refined foods that are low in nutrients. Others contend that the overuse of antibiotics triggers serious imbalance in the intestinal ecology, resulting in inflammation and susceptibility to parasitic invasion. Yet others believe that toxic substances in the environment disrupt the metabolic machinery required to metabolize dietary macro and micronutrients. It is my opinion that the interplay of these and other factors probably contribute to the increasing incidence of food allergy in contemporary society.

How might this occur? Ours is an overconsumptive society. We know that overconsumption can lead to the development of food intolerance. This can occur when foods are consumed in large amounts or with high frequency. When overconsumption of refined foods occurs, a situation of high caloric intake coupled with low nutrient density exists. The result is insufficient nutrients to metabolize the ingested calories. The body must then rely on its reserves of these nutrients to drive the enzymes needed to metabolize such foods. Obviously, this cannot continue for long or the body's nutrient reserves will be depleted—especially in the case of water-soluble nutrients.

Added to this is the overconsumption of antibiotics. Whether our antibiotics are consumed for therapeutic reasons or through the food supply, the effects on digestion and metabolism can be significant. Inflammation, parasitic infestation, and food allergy have been linked to antibiotic overuse. Antibiotic use is linked to the so-called "leaky gut syndrome." In this syndrome, the intestinal lining has become thin and porous due to inflammation. The increased porosity of the gut leads to an increased uptake of incompletely digested proteins (or IBPs, discussed in chapter 5). The IBPs are absorbed intact and reacted upon by circulating lymphocytes in the blood. Thus, an allergic response to foods can occur from antibiotic overuse. Until the intestinal integrity is restored, reactivity to foods continues.

How does one restore intestinal integrity? This is a complex issue that is not fully understood. We do know that nutrients such as vitamin A, beta-carotene, zinc, folic acid, vitamin E, and essential fatty acids are all vital to the rebuilding of the intestinal mucosa. Unfortunately, when intestinal inflammation exists, there is often reduced absorption of nutrients. Feeding a diet already low in nutrients will not encourage intestinal healing or reduction of food allergies. Therefore, some form of nutritional supplementation and dietary change is needed.

Then there is the problem of intestinal bacteria. When the colon is overrun with coliform bacteria or parasites such as *Candida albicans* or *Giardia lamblia*, these organisms must be dealt with before any restoration of intestinal integrity can occur. This usually involves anti-parasitic agents, nutrients, and reinoculation of the bowel with *Lactobacilli*. Food allergy occurs with great frequency when intestinal lactobacillus levels are low.

Heavy metals, such as lead and mercury, are yet another factor that may interfere with proper metabolism and contribute to the development of food allergy. Lead is commonly found in the food, water, and air in the United States. Lead binds strongly with enzymes throughout the body. When lead binds with digestive enzymes, the enzymes become inactivated. In this state, the enzymes cannot carry out their task of breaking down food properly. The result is impaired digestion, impaired absorption, and development of food allergy. Lead has also been shown to have an adverse effect upon immune function.

When dietary fiber intake is low, the transit of food through the digestive tract is slowed. When this occurs, partially digested food resides in the intestine for much longer than normal. This creates an environment in which intestinal bacteria can begin to putrefy the contents of the intestine. As this occurs, the pH of the gut changes, which results in an environment that often favors the growth of pathogenic bacteria at the expense of *Lactobacilli* and other beneficial organisms. One consequence is the development of food intolerance.

The above discussion only touches on the complexity of what must be considered in the management of allergy. The management of airborne allergy often requires changes in the child's immediate environment to reduce exposure to the offending agents. This is a beginning. Nutritional status also must be carefully evaluated. I've observed a direct link between the severity of airborne allergy and the presence of food allergy. When food allergy is properly managed, problems with airborne allergy frequently improve.

The management of food allergy (or hypersensitivity) begins with the identification of offenders. No matter which approach is taken, it is always helpful to reduce the intake of offending foods for a time. At the very least, foods should be rotated. This is especially true in pan-sensitive individuals who react adversely to nearly everything they eat. Often, simply removing cow's milk from the diet is enough to significantly reduce the occurrence of otitis media.

In food-allergic individuals, the intestinal function must be evaluated. This involves understanding bowel transit times, possible parasitic infection, nutritional status, enzyme activity, stool composition, absorption, and much more. The diet must be carefully evaluated to detect any significant imbalances in macronutrient or micronutrient intake.

Methods of Allergy Testing[7]

The methods described below are currently used to identify allergy to various substances.

Skin Testing (scratch test): Used to identify IgE-mediated reactions. The skin is pricked with a "scarifier" through a drop of antigen-containing solution. The skin is then observed for the development of characteristic reactions that include varying degrees of swelling and redness.

Radioallergosorbent Test (RAST): IgE-RAST detects antigen-specific IgE, type I immediate hypersensitivity. IgG RAST detects delayed sensitivity reactions.

Intradermal Cutaneous Test: Used to identify immediate hypersensitivity reactions. The antigen is injected into the superficial layers of skin. The skin is observed for characteristic reactions.

Food Immune Complex Assay (FICA): Used to identify both immediate and delayed reactivity.

Elimination-Provocation: Used to identify food allergy and hypersensitivity, i.e., food intolerance. (Allergy and hypersensitivity cannot be differentiated using this test.) Performed by putting the patient on an oligo-antigenic diet for one week, then challenging, one at a time, with suspected food antigens. A simplified version of this test can be done at home.

Sublingual Provocation: Detects hypersensitivity reaction. Suspected foods are placed under the tongue, then the deltoid or other major muscle group is tested for strength. Muscle response is measured manually or with instrumentation. Weakening of the muscle upon challenge with a food indicates sensitivity to the test item.

Of the above tests, elimination-provocation (EP) is the most reliable since it identifies both allergy and hypersensitivity (although it does not differentiate). Its chief drawbacks are that it: 1) takes days to weeks to complete, 2) requires patient motivation and compliance, potentially limiting the number of foods that can be tested, 3) does not give a clear indication of the degree of reactivity, and 4) is difficult to test for reactivity to additives and chemicals found in food (although, thus far, no tests are particularly successful at this). In spite of these drawbacks, EP is one of the most acceptable, reliable, and cost-effective assessment tools available for identifying food intolerance. It is advisable to use some form of EP in conjunction with laboratory tests.

Homeopathic Medicine

There are two basic considerations in the homeopathic management of otitis media. First, acute otitis media is managed using remedies that are selected based on their similarity to the acute syndrome. (See chapter 6.) While some of these remedies may be useful in chronic otitis media, they are specifically useful in acute otitis media. Second, chronic otitis media is believed to arise out of a fundamental weakness in the child's constitution or out of suppressive therapeutic intervention. In these cases, the homeopathic remedy is selected after an extensive evaluation of the complete symptom picture of the child. During the course of constitutional care, an acute flare-up of otitis media may occur. The doctor may then choose to treat the acute episode with an "acute" remedy and resume constitutional care once the episode has subsided.

Stephen Messer, N.D., has extensive experience in the homeopathic management of otitis media. At a 1986 conference on homeopathic medicine, he presented a lecture entitled "Homeopathy and Otitis in Children." In his address, Dr. Messer described in detail the process of decision-making that goes into selecting the appropriate remedy.* The following diagnostic categories form a basis for Messer's approach.[8]

Otitis Media Without Effusion: Redness of the tympanic membrane with normal mobility. There is no fluid.

Acute Otitis Media: Same signs as above. In addition, there is suppuration in the middle ear, and decreased mobility of the tympanic membrane.

Otitis Media With Effusion: Serous fluid or pus lies behind the tympanic membrane. Mobility of the tympanic membrane is limited. There is often an absence of other symptoms.

Chronic Otitis Media: Chronic discharge of fluid, often pus, from the middle ear.

---

*An audio tape of this lecture is available through Homeopathic Educational Services. See resources.

You diagnose acute otitis media in a child.

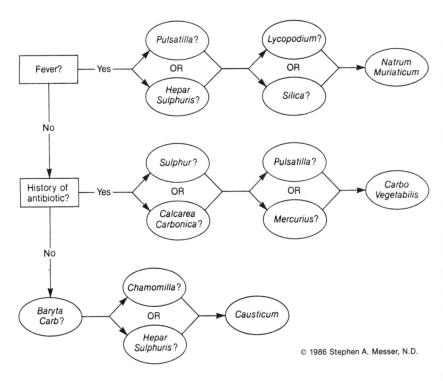

© 1986 Stephen A. Messer, N.D.

Figure 15
Acute Otitis Media

In otitis media without effusion and acute otitis media, the process of remedy selection is rather straightforward (although it still requires an evaluation of the child's general symptom pattern). First, a diagnosis of the child's condition is made based on otoscopic findings. Once the diagnosis is made, you refer to the appropriate flow chart (figures 15, 16, and 17).[9] For example, if you diagnose otitis media without effusion, the first question you ask is, is there a fever of more than 103 degrees? If the answer is "yes", you go to the next level of questioning. In this case, is the face bright red? If the

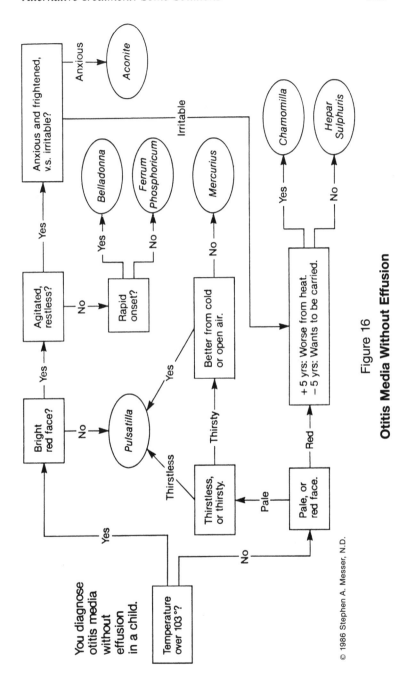

Figure 16
Otitis Media Without Effusion

© 1986 Stephen A. Messer, N.D.

Figure 17
Chronic or Recurrent Otitis Media

answer is "no", the remedy is *Pulsatilla*. If the answer is "yes", you determine if the child is agitated and restless. Using this progression of logic, the correct remedy can be selected. The same type of process is used in acute otitis media. These flow diagrams are especially useful in small children, since small children can rarely communicate specifics about their pain.

In otitis media with effusion and chronic otitis media, Messer has observed that there is a hierarchy of remedies that must be considered. Remedies listed at the top of the hierarchy are those more commonly used in chronic otitis media. Those at the bottom are less frequently used, but no less important. Since chronic otitis media requires constitutional care, the hierarchy should be considered as a guide. The doctor must then research the *materia medica* for the remedies that fit the individual child.

Otitis media with effusion and chronic otitis media often occur as a result of repeated doses of antibiotics or because of an underlying constitutional weakness. In either case, remedies are required that are deep acting and can stir a response in a suppressed immune system. Occasionally, a child treated for chronic otitis media may get worse for a period before improving. This is because: 1) chronic otitis media often occurs with only minimal symptomatology, thus any change tends to appear as an aggravation, and 2) a deep-acting remedy frequently arouses the body defenses sufficiently to begin acting against an ongoing infection. This type of response is not cause for alarm, but should be monitored closely. Communication with the parents of such a child is important.

The remedies described below are those most frequently used in chronic otitis media or otitis media with effusion. Recognize that remedy selection is not-clear cut in these children. When ear discharge occurs, the type of discharge is an important indicator in remedy selection. However, children with chronic otitis are frequently asymptomatic, so ear signs and symptoms may be of limited value. In addition, silent forms of otitis media such as these may harbor complications. It is necessary to be alert for signs of meningitis, mastoiditis, and other potential problems. Anytime complications are threatening or present, a specialist should be consulted.

Dosage and Potencies

A method of prescribing known as Kent's Scale of Ascending Potencies is a useful means of regulating the dosage of homeopathic remedies.[10] In acute otitis media, the chosen remedy is given once every hour to four hours depending upon the severity of the child's condition. The remedy is continued until progress stalls. At this point, the initial remedy is discontinued and replaced by the same remedy at the next higher potency. Thus, if *Pulsatilla* 12x worked initially, but symptoms reappeared after 36 to 48 hours, *Pulsatilla* 30x would be given next. Obviously, if there is no improvement in the child's condition within this period, the wrong remedy was chosen. In this situation, a reevaluation of the case is required.

Constitutional care often requires the prescription of higher potencies (200x to 1M)* since they are deeper-acting. These dosages are given infrequently. Often, the prescriber gives one dose of the high-potency remedy, and observes progress for the next three to eight weeks before prescribing again.

Remedies Used in Chronic Otitis Media and Otitis Media with Effusion

The following remedies are listed in alphabetical order for easy reference. This is not an order of their frequency of use in otitis media. Also, this is an abbreviated *materia medica*. It may be necessary to consult a complete *materia medica*. For remedies used in acute otitis media and otitis media without effusion, refer to chapter 6.

It is important to note that a child need not display all the symptoms of a medicine in order for that medicine to be effective.

Baryta carbonica

In this child, the tonsils are almost always swollen. When colds occur, which they do frequently, they usually begin as a sore throat. Cold air affects his tonsils adversely. When otorrhea occurs, it is often bloody. This child is physically shorter than other children his age and is often described as dwarfish. He is slow to develop and is usually behind his peers in learning to walk and talk, in gaining weight, and in most other areas.[11] If he tries to exert himself, he becomes very tired and weak to the point of feeling exhausted. This child has poor posture, commonly a lumbar lordosis, coupled with a hard, distended abdomen. He tends to salivate heavily.

Emotionally, the *Baryta carb* child is touchy and irritable. He does not like to be interfered with. There is a fear of being left alone, going out of doors, or being around strangers.

---

*Only an experienced homeopath should consider prescribing potencies in this range.

Excessive shyness is a characteristic of the *Baryta carb* child. Nightmares are common.

Mentally, this child is inattentive, forgetful, and has a short attention span. He may play with an object for one moment, then drop it and move on to something else. If he learns a new task or verse, he may forget it within a few hours or by the next day. He is often not sure he is doing the right thing.

This is one of the grand remedies for use in children with Down syndrome (although its use is by no means restricted to such children).

Symptoms are worse: from washing, bathing, and lying down.

Symptoms are better: from open air.

Calcarea carbonica

Calcarea is commonly used as a constitutional medicine. There is a tendency toward collections of fluid in various parts of the body including the middle ear. There is a thick, muco-purulent discharge from the middle ear, enlarged lymph nodes, and swollen tonsils. Recurrent infections and excessive production of mucus in the respiratory tract are important physical signs.

The *Calcarea* child is thirsty and prefers cold drinks. He craves indigestible things to eat such as chalk, pencils, or dirt. He also craves salt, eggs, raw potatoes, and sweets. Milk disagrees with him. There is usually a definite dislike of hot food, with a craving for cold things like ice cream.

Physically, the child in need of *Calcarea* is soft, plump, fair-skinned, and lethargic. He is often overweight. He is weak, easily tired, and content to just sit around doing nothing. The *Calcarea* child is sluggish in movement and does poorly at games. The slightest exertion causes him to sweat. He may have head sweats during sleep. Mentally, this child is slow and may have difficulty in school. He often lacks the motivation to persevere in mental tasks. Fearfulness and apprehension are common *Calcarea* traits. After *Baryta carb*, this is the most commonly indicated remedy for children with Down syndrome (although its use is by no means restricted to such children).

While the above signs accurately describe the *Calcarea* child, recognize that this medicine is used commonly for various complaints of infancy.

Symptoms are worse: from cold, damp weather, and mental or physical exertion.

Symptoms are better: from dry weather, lying down on the painful side, and warmth.

Calcarea sulphuricum

The *Calcarea sulph* child typically displays mucus discharges that are yellow, thick, and lumpy. There is often a discharge of yellow matter from the eyes. Otorrhea is thick, muco-purulent, and bloody. Pimples and pustules on the face are not uncommon. The soles of the feet burn and itch. There are no marked emotional signs that indicate *Calcarea sulph*.

Capsicum

This remedy is useful when the inflammation has spread to the mastoid process and there is chronic suppuration of the tympanic membrane, accompanied by bursting headache and chilliness. There are burning and stinging pains in the ear, which extend to the throat. There is great swelling and pain behind ears. This remedy is also useful in the perforation of the membrane with purulent discharge. The ear is tender to touch.[12] When coughing occurs, painful symptoms are often experienced in distant parts of the body such as the legs or ears. There is much thirst, but drinking causes this child to shiver. This remedy suits plethoric, sluggish, cold, and weak children with diminished vital heat.

Symptoms are worse: from uncovering, drafts, and open air.

Symptoms are better: while eating and from heat.

Carbo vegetabilis

The typical *Carbo* child is sluggish, overweight, and lazy. He seems to have never fully recovered from the effects of some previous illness. The body is almost bluish and is icy-cold. The face is pale. Emotionally he fears the dark. Nosebleeds are common.

Any overindulgence causes headaches. The child experiences contractive pain in the abdomen. Eructations, heaviness, and fullness are characteristic digestive signs. Digestion is slow. The child is averse to milk, meat, and fat. He is distressed by the simplest foods. This remedy is sometimes used for children with intestinal colic. The abdomen is often greatly distended. A dry cough with hoarseness that worsens in the evening accompanies wheezing with rattling of mucus in the chest. This child is cold from the knees down to the feet. The skin is a cold blue, but perspiration is hot.

Symptoms are worse: from cold, fat food, butter, milk, warm damp weather, open air, and in evening.

Symptoms are better: from eructation and fanning.

Hepar sulphuricum

Hepar sulph is generally not used in the early stages of an earache. It is used when symptoms have progressed and pus has formed in the middle ear. There is frequently a nasal discharge that is at first watery, then becomes thick, yellow, and offensive. There is intense throbbing pain in the ear, accompanied by diminished hearing. These children are irritable and sensitive. Like the *Chamomilla* child, the *Hepar* child is cross and easily angered. They can be provoked to a tantrum with little effort. A hallmark of the *Hepar* child is oversensitivity to touch, cold, and pain. The cold sensitivity may be so great that even a hand or foot exposed from beneath the covers results in aggravation of symptoms.

Symptoms are worse: from dry cold winds, cold foods, touch, pressure, night, exertion, or the slightest draft.

Symptoms are better: from warmth, extra clothing or covers, humidity, hot applications, and after eating.

Hydrastis

Hydrastis has an especially strong action on the mucous membranes. This remedy is characterized by secretions that are thick, yellowish, and ropy regardless of which area of the body is involved. There is roaring in the ears, hearing loss, and a chronic muco-purulent discharge. Eustachian catarrh is common. There is a thick mucus secretion that runs from the nasopharynx down the back of the throat. Meanwhile, a watery secretion is discharged through the nares. This child is weak, has poor digestion, and suffers from constipation. There may be a dry, harsh cough that progresses to bronchial catarrh in later stages.

Kali bichromicum

Children in need of this remedy typically have a tough, stringy, viscous discharge from the mucous membranes. What distinguishes the discharge of *Kali bic* is its sticky, gluey quality. Whether the discharge is from the nose, ears, or lungs, it has this distinctive quality.

Another characteristic of this remedy is pains that migrate quickly. The pain may be in one area, then move to another. At another point the pain may be gone. This child is usually worse in the morning. From 2 A.M. to 3 A.M., most symptoms are aggravated. He is better from heat, but hot weather makes him worse. *Kali bic* should never be used when there is fever.

Symptoms are worse: from hot weather, undressing, cold, from 2 A.M. to 3 A.M., and in the morning.

Symptoms are better: from warmth.

Lycopodium

A characteristic of this remedy is symptoms that are on or begin on the right side. There may be a humming and roaring sensation in the ear with diminished hearing. A thick, yellow, offensive discharge is common. The nose is stopped up. There is often a viscous and offensive perspiration, especially on the feet and axillae. *Lycopodium* is especially indicated in the child with digestive complaints such as gas and bloating. Digestion is poor and irregular. Eating the tiniest amount causes fullness. The child is thin and weak. He often has cold hands and feet. Symptoms are aggravated between 4 to 8 P.M. or from 4 P.M. to midnight.

The *Lycopodium* child is fearful, apprehensive, and afraid to be alone. Sometimes the child wants to be alone, but needs to have someone nearby or in the next room. He is averse to taking on new things. He can be headstrong and scornful when sick. Fright, anger, or embarrassment may likely bring on illness. This is a remedy that may be used at any stage of an earache.

Symptoms are worse: from lying on the right side, heat or a warm room, hot air, cold food or drink, eating, and from 4 P.M. to 8 P.M.

Symptoms are better: from warm food and drink, being uncovered, cool or open air, motion, and after midnight.

Mercurius

Mercurius is indicated when there is pus formation and is often used in more chronic cases of otitis media. The nasal discharge is yellow-green and offensive (as are all body secretions in these children). There is profuse, offensive perspiration. Lymph nodes are chronically swollen. Tonsils are swollen and may be covered with pockets of pus and open sores. The gums are soft, swollen, and bleed easily. There is great thirst. The skin is almost constantly moist. If the skin is consistently dry, *Mercurius* is not the remedy. Increased salivation, bad breath, and puffiness of the tongue are general *Mercurius* symptoms.

The child in need of *Mercurius* is often described as a human "thermometer" because she is acutely sensitive to heat, cold, and nearly all environmental influences. The *Mercurius* child is weak and may tire at the slightest exertion. There is sometimes muscular trembling. This child seems to display a loss of will-power. She is agitated, hurried, impulsive, and has difficulty concentrating.

Symptoms are worse: from damp, cold, rainy weather, heat, sweating, motion, exertion, open air, lying on the right side, at night, and in a warm bed or warm room.

Symptoms are better: in moderate temperatures.

Natrum muriaticum

Natrum mur is indicated when there is great weakness and weariness. The mental signs are perhaps the most useful in this child because emotional events are often what precipitates illness in him. This is the child who becomes ill when there is fighting between parents, a public scolding, or loss of a family member or anyone close to him. If he is brought to anger, he may become ill because he is easily angered, but does not freely express his feelings. The *Natrum mur* child is irritable and is infuriated by seemingly trivial things. He rarely cries in public, but may cry alone. Any attempts to console him may be met with anger. He is oversensitive to stimulus and easily startled.

The child awakens with much sneezing. Heavy nasal discharge, described as having a raw egg-white appearance, is present. Small eruptions or vesicles form around the lips. The lips and corners of the mouth are dry, ulcerated, and cracked. A crack in the middle of the lower lip is sometimes seen.

Symptoms are worse: from noise, consolation, lying down, heat, talking, and in a warm room.

Symptoms are better: from cold bathing, lying on right side, going without regular meals, and in open air.

Psorinum

The child in need of *Psorinum* is extremely sensitive to cold. He wants his head kept warm and wants warm clothing even in summer. The child catches cold easily. Weakness persists long after recovery. All body secretions have an offensive smell. Emotionally, this child is melancholy with feelings of hopelessness and despair. There are frequently red, raw, oozing scabs around the ears that release an offensive discharge. This is accompanied by intense itching. The face also may contain skin eruptions. There is chronic, offensive otorrhea of a brownish color. There is great swelling of the tonsils with painful swallowing.

The *Psorinum* child is always hungry and desires to eat in the middle of the night. He experiences hay fever, which returns irregularly every year. The hallmark of this child is problems with the skin. There is intolerable itching that often keeps him awake at night. Eruptions occur on the scalp and at the bends of joints. Exertion causes urticaria.

Symptoms are worse: from changes of weather, cold, and the slightest draft.

Symptoms are better: from heat, warm clothing, and in summer.

Pulsatilla

Pulsatilla is not commonly indicated in chronic otitis media. However, when the constitutional picture is that of *Pulsatilla*, the healing response can be dramatic even in chronic otitis media. *Pulsatilla* is suitable for almost all types of ear pain. The child who needs *Pulsatilla* is gentle, weepy, sensitive, and loves to be held. He desires attention and is easily consoled by a sympathetic response. The *Pulsatilla* child is sometimes described as moody because he can be happy one moment and profoundly sad the next. He often feels sorry for himself and laments his plight during illness.

The cheeks are pale. He feels better when in open, fresh air. There is a thick, bland, yellowish-green nasal discharge. The eardrum is swollen and red, with fluid. If the ear is draining, the discharge is usually thick and yellowish-green. The ear is swollen, red, and hot, and there is deep itching in it. The pain often goes through the whole side of the face. There may be a stopped sensation in the ear. A dry or loose cough can be present. Symptoms often come on gradually and frequently follow a cold. The child may be feverish, but show a surprising absence of thirst.

Symptoms are worse: from heat, lying down, exertion, after eating, toward evening, and in a warm room.

Symptoms are better: with motion, cold applications, cold food and drink, and in open air.

Silica

According to Randall Neustaedter, C.A., *Silica* is the most frequently indicated constitutional remedy for chronic otitis media. He reports that, of 21 cases of chronic or recurrent otitis media, 43 percent responded favorably to treatment with *Silica*.[13] The child in need of *Silica* is likely to experience discharge from the ear. He is sensitive and anxious. *Silica* is often indicated when a cold or bronchial condition is long-standing or slow to respond. Symptoms are severe. There is often roaring in the ears, and the child is sensitive to noise. The *Silica* child is cold, chilly, and wants plenty of warm clothing. He hates drafts, and his hands and feet are icy cold. There is offensive sweat on the hands, feet, and axillae. *Silica* is the remedy most often required when there is pain behind the ear on the mastoid process. (See also *Hepar sulph*) Repair of the tympanic membrane can more often be achieved with *Silica* than with any other remedy.[14]

Emotionally this child is yielding, faint-hearted, and anxious. He is nervous, excitable, and sensitive, but can be obstinate. The *Silica* child tends to be weak and is easily exhausted.

Symptoms are worse: from cold, open air, winter, damp weather, cold food or drink, lying on the painful side, eating, and in morning.

Symptoms are better: from warmth.

Sulphur

Sulphur is especially indicated when there is an extensive history of antibiotic use. It has an exceptional ability to arouse the bodily defenses when they have been suppressed due to long-standing illness or drugs. The mucous membranes are characteristically hot, dry, and red. The mouth and lips may burn. There may be redness around the anus with itching. Most *Sulphur* children have constipation, although they may sometimes awaken with diarrhea. The *Sulphur* child urinates copious amounts of colorless urine. There is frequent urination with eneuresis. Burning of the hands, soles of the feet, and top of the head is common.

Breathing is sometimes difficult, and the child feels better when the window is open or when out of doors. The skin is dry, scaly, and unhealthy. Every injury tends to open and become infected. The skin itches and burns. Scratching or bathing irritates the skin immensely, but bathing aggravates nearly all symptoms. All body discharges are offensive, especially perspiration.

The *Sulphur* child is quite thirsty and drinks much liquid, although milk causes digestive upset. He is very weak and faint around 11 A.M. and must have something to eat. The *Sulphur* child has a well-developed appetite with very definite taste preferences. Yet, he becomes sluggish and tired after meals. Cold weather and fresh air invigorate the *Sulphur* child. Emotionally, the child is self-centered and demanding. He is often overconcerned with possessions and may take great pride in his toys, which he often hoards.

Symptoms are worse: from bathing, washing, cold air, warmth, standing, scratching, at 11 A.M., and on the left side.

Symptoms are better: from dry, warm weather; lying on right side, open air, and warm drinks.

Tellurium

Tellurium is not a common remedy in otitis media, but when the constitutional picture matches, it can be invaluable. There is eczema behind the ear and middle ear catarrh that may drain outward. Otorrhea is acrid, often described as smelling like "fish-pickle." It is watery, but frequently excoriating (tending to abrade the surrounding skin). There is intense itching, swelling, and throbbing in the ear canal. The child in need of *Tellurium* has a very sensitive back. Pain usually runs from the seventh cervical vertebra to the fifth thoracic. These children are very sensitive to touch. Even the friction of clothing may be bothersome. There may be sacral and sciatic pains.

This remedy is characterized by circular patches (like ringworm) on the skin, accompanied by itching. Emotionally the child is neglectful and forgetful. The action of this remedy may take long to develop.

Symptoms are worse: from coughing, laughing, touch, lying on the painful side, while at rest at night, and in cold weather.

Symptoms are better: The coryza, lachrymation, and hoarseness are better in open air.

Manipulation

When otitis media is due to dysfunctional mechanics in the upper cervical spine, manual manipulation of the affected vertebrae should be considered an essential part of treatment. According to Gutmann, ". . . in this syndrome [occipito-atlanto-axial joint dysfunction] the success of adjustment overshadows every other type of treatment, especially the pharmaceutical approach. . . ."[15]

Spinal Problems

A. History: The history will frequently, but not always, contain incidences of trauma to the head or neck.

    1. Trauma (macrotrauma or microtrauma)

        a. Birth
- Vacuum extraction
- Forceps
- Cesarean section
- Prolonged or difficult vaginal delivery
- Normal birth*
- First child

        b. Other injuries
- Rough play with peers
- Falls from changing table, bed, down stairs, etc.
- Overzealous play by parents (throwing or spinning the child)
- Physical abuse by caregiver

    2. General

The following generalized signs have been found to be associated with upper cervical biomechanical dysfunction. Some of these signs may indicate more serious disease, so the physician should proceed with the full spectrum of diagnostic possibilities in mind.

- Lowered resistance to infection of the ear, nose, and throat
- Conjunctivitis
- Sleeping difficulty
- Neck pain, stiffness, or rigidity
- Headaches
- Torticollis (especially infantile)

---

*Strong uterine contractions may contribute to musculoskeletal injury even during a delivery which is considered normal or uneventful.

— Seizures
— Vomiting
— Hyperactivity
— Morphological deformations of the bony skeleton
— Intestinal colic

B. Examination

   1. Palpation

      a. Motion palpation of the occipito-atlanto-axial complex

        — Observe for abnormal relational movement of the vertebrae on flexion, extension, right and left rotation, and lateral flexion.

      b. Static palpation of the occipito-atlanto-axial complex

      c. Palpation of soft tissue

        — Note areas of swelling, muscle spasm and rigidity, areas of muscle hypotonicity, heat, and tenderness.

        — Note "feel" and tenderness of local acupoints.

   2. Radiographic

      a. X-ray analysis is used by some to establish proper line of drive and contact, not to establish mechanical relationships.

      b. In cases of trauma, X-ray should be considered to rule out fracture, dislocation, instability of atlanto-axial ligament, basilar invagination, etc.

      c. There is a high incidence of atlanto-axial instability in children with Down syndrome due to laxity of the transverse atlantal ligament, or anomalous axis formation. Since this is a high-risk group for otitis media, it is important to know that upper cervical manipulation in these children can result in fatal consequences. For a review of the chiropractic evaluation and management of the Down syndrome child refer to "A Chiropractic Perspective in Atlanto-axial Instability in Down's Syndrome."[16]

— Note that when the initial bout of otitis media begins early in life, for example at 0-5 months, functional problems of the cervical spine should be considered.

C. Mechanical Findings

In otitis media, a number of possible structural relationships may occur in the cervical spine. The most common biomechanical contributor to otitis media is atlanto-occipital dysfunction (or subluxation).

1. Occiput. It is more common to find the side of subluxation on the same side as the middle ear involvement. However, this does not always occur. Bilateral otitis media often occurs with bilateral occipital involvement.

   a. Anterior right, left, or bilateral
   b. Posterior right, left, or bilateral
   c. Lateral right or left

2. 1st Cervical (C1, also known as the atlas). Subluxation of C1 occurs frequently in otitis media. Like occipital involvement, C1 involvement is commonly on the same side as the middle ear problem. Bilateral otitis media often occurs with bilateral C1 involvement.

   a. Anterior right, left, or bilateral
   b. Posterior right, left, or bilateral
   c. Lateral right or left

3. 2nd Cervical (C2, also known as the axis). Subluxation of C2 is present less frequently in otitis media than is subluxation of C1 or occiput. When this occurs, it is usually posterior or lateral. Anteriority is less common, but does occur.

    a. Anterior right, left, or bilateral
    b. Posterior right, left, or bilateral
    c. Lateral right or left

4. Thoracic mobilization may be indicated, especially when there is respiratory congestion. Thoracic mobilization has been shown to enhance immune function.

In acute otitis media, if biomechanical involvement is a chief contributor, symptoms should abate within 24 hours following treatment. If they do not, other factors are responsible. Even when biomechanical problems are believed to be present in acute otitis media, it is necessary to address dietary and nutritional factors as well. Homeopathic care, acupuncture, and allergy management are vital adjuncts that should be considered in the overall management. It is my opinion that only a small percentage of children with otitis media due to biomechanical problems require manipulation alone. The majority of cases require adjunctive care as well.

In chronic otitis media, manipulation can only be considered one aspect of the treatment plan. In these children, the degree of constitutional weakness and middle ear inflammation is significant. The overall strategy *must* involve assessment and management of diet, food allergy, and nutrition. I've found that homeopathic medicine, acupuncture, and botanical medicine are the most successful means of restoring a child with constitutional weakness to optimum health. Children with acute or chronic otitis media may require antibiotic intervention at various stages. Under these circumstances, it is still important to manage biomechanical problems.

The above discussion only represents guidelines. The clinician should conduct a customary physical examination to determine the precise state of cervical biomechanics. It is assumed that those engaging in manipulative therapy have had prior professional training in manipulation. Those without training should not attempt manipulation of the cervical spine, especially in children.

Temperomandibular Joint Problems

Temperomandibular joint (TMJ) dysfunction, while not proven to be a cause of recurrent otitis media in children, is a suspected contributor. In adults, TMJ dysfunction often results in symptoms of ear pain, fullness of the ear, and sometimes hearing deficit.

Unfortunately, the causes of TMJ problems are many and management is complex. Bruxism* is often a cause of TMJ dysfunction in children (although it can be a result of TMJ dysfunction as well). Bruxism can be brought on by parasites, allergies, emotional stress, or other factors. TMJ problems also can develop in children who are bottlefed from infancy. The nutritional inadequacy of formula, coupled with the reduced sucking associated with bottlefeeding results in potential malformation of the jaw, cranial bones, and bite. There are presently no universally accepted means of diagnosis and treatment of TMJ dysfunction.

Articular Strains of the Cranium

Trauma at birth contributes to articular strains in the newborn cranium that persist into childhood unless corrective steps are taken. Normal pelvic forces cause great shifting of the cranial bones as the child emerges from the birth canal. When forceps are used, the resulting strains can be significant.

When examining the newborn, infant, toddler, or older child with otitis media, facial symmetry should be considered. Careful observation often reveals asymmetry in the maxillae, zygomatic arches, temporal bones, parietal bones, and other less conspicuous cranial structures. Cranial asymmetry suggests fixation of the sutures at some location. In some children with otitis media, it may be necessary to correct this fixation before progress can occur.

---

*Bruxism is defined as grinding of the teeth, especially during sleep.

The role of cranial manipulation in managing otitis media is not clearly established. However, numerous clinical accounts suggest that it can be of great value.

Acupuncture

Material in this section (except where noted) was reprinted from *The Treatment of Children by Acupuncture*, by Julian Scott, Ph.D., published by the Journal of Chinese Medicine. (Please note that the original manuscript was formatted in a way that might provide added meaning.) Dr. Scott's book is the definitive work on pediatric acupuncture, and I highly recommend it for anyone who treats children. The format is clear and concise.

This section contains a very specialized vocabulary which may seem technical to those unfamiliar with acupuncture. However, since this chapter is intended for practitioners I have assumed prior knowledge of terms. For more information on acupuncture see the suggested reading section of the appendices.

*   *   *

Otitis media is common among children of all ages, and those who are prone may have repeated attacks. It causes great distress, and for many conditions (especially viral in origin), there is no treatment in Western medicine. Acupuncture offers a cure both in the acute phase and as a preventive against repeated attacks. In Western medicine, otitis is always regarded as being due to external attack of viral or bacterial origin. In Chinese medicine, some conditions are regarded as due to external pathogenic wind and others as due to internal heat flaring up in the liver channel.

This approach helps to explain why some children are more prone to attacks than others. If internal heat (either Ji-heat or liver heat) already exists, then it is easy for external pathogenic factors to enter. The cause of heat in very young children is Ji-blockage, while in children of seven years and above, the heat may be due to emotional causes, especially emotional tension generated by trying to please over-ambitious parents.

Regarding external pathogenic factors, it is easy for any upper respiratory tract infection to spread to the ears and cause otitis. Once established, it may return frequently in the syndrome of 'pathogenic factor remaining.' Another common cause is water in the ear from too much swimming. This is especially common among children who swim as a spare-time activity in the evening and who are thus prone to being over-tired.

As far as the differentiation of syndromes is concerned, the main distinctions presented here are as follows:

i) Non-purulent, or catarrhal, as opposed to purulent. The catarrhal type often has little or no discharge from the ear or nose, and if there is any discharge it is clear and watery. By contrast, the purulent type always has a thick yellow discharge, often foul-smelling. The purulent type is basically similar to the catarrhal, but it has the additional complication of damp building up in the body.

ii) Acute as opposed to chronic. Here chronic means more or less continuous earache, usually with discharge. Chronic otitis may have periods of acute attack.

iii) External cause as opposed to internal. The external cause is wind or damp obstructing the ear cavities, and the internal cause is liver-heat or damp heat in the liver entering the channel and causing obstruction. In practice, many acute attacks have both an internal and an external factor. It is then for the practitioner to decide on the emphasis of treatment.

In carrying out a diagnosis on a child with an acute attack or with recurrent attacks, the ear area should be palpated for tenderness and for swollen glands. The otoscope is useful in determining the severity of the condition and in assessing the progress of treatment.

Etiology and Pathology

A. Acute catarrhal

1. Etiology

   External pathogenic wind, either in the form of an infection which spreads to the ear or cold wind blowing on the ear; or damp pathogenic factor from damp weather or too much swimming; or heat which affects the liver and gall bladder channels.

2. Pathology

   The ear cavity receives jing from the kidneys and yang qi from the channels. Jing and yang together allow hearing to take place. If there is invasion of pathogenic heat, wind, or damp, it can block the qi and cause obstruction. The obstruction enters the cavities, giving rise to deafness and a distending or bursting sensation in the ear.

   The most common cause is external pathogenic wind which blocks up the ear cavities so that the inside and outside become unregulated. The other main cause is liver and gall bladder oppressed heat which enters the channels and rises up to the ear cavities, causing the qi to knot and the jing-luo to become stuck and obstructed, giving rise to otitis media.

B. Acute Purulent

1. Etiology

   Invasion of external pathogenic wind-heat poison, often originating in the respiratory tract and rising up to the ear due to excessively spicy, heating, or damp-producing foods; or Ji-heat causing heat and damp in the liver and gall bladder channels.

2. Pathology

   The zheng-qi cannot resist the pathogenic factor of wind-heat/damp-poison. The pathogenic factor passes to the eardrum and then to the middle ear, where it causes stagnation of fluid. The stagnant fluid transforms to pus which is discharged through the external ear. Alternatively, liver and gall bladder damp-heat enters the channels and rises up, penetrating the ear cavities where it collects and transforms into pus.

C. Chronic catarrhal

   1. Etiology

The result of acute otitis media which is not cured or only partially cured (pathogenic factor remaining), or the body is feeble and weak from overwork or long-term disease.

   2. Pathology

The pathogenic factor remains and is not cleared, blocking up the ear cavities so that the qi and blood are stuck and obstructed; or the body is weak and the liver and kidney jing are insufficient; or the spleen qi is xu and weak, so that the jing is without the support necessary to send it up. The ear cavity is then without nourishment.

Otitis media

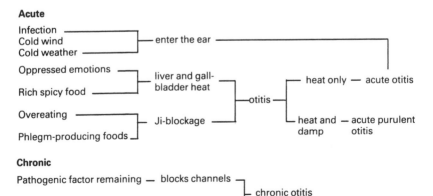

Clinical Manifestations and Differentiation of Syndromes

A. Acute catarrhal

    1. Pathogenic wind enters the cavities

        — Ear stuffed up, hearing power reduced
        — Tinnitus
        — Mild ear pain
        — Ear drum bleeding slightly
        — Occasional upper respiratory tract infection
        — Dislikes cold
        — Fever
        — Headache
        — Nasal discharge

        Pulse: floating

        Treatment principle: Expel wind and clear heat, regulate the ear cavity, and drain damp.

    2. Liver and gall bladder oppressed heat

        — Inner ear distended and full, bleeding from eardrum, fluid in ear passage
        — Dizziness
        — Headache with swollen feeling, pressure, and bursting sensation
        — Buzzing in ears, hearing power reduced

        Tongue: body red
        Tongue coat: yellow
        Pulse: wiry or slippery, rapid

        Treatment principle: Clear liver and gall bladder heat, resolve damp, and regulate the ear cavity.

B. Acute purulent

    1. Wind-heat at the superficial level

        Before the purulent stage, there are the symptoms and signs characteristic of wind-heat:

— Uncomfortable body
— Dislikes wind
— Chills and maybe fevers
— Headache

followed by:

— Earache and ear pain
— Hearing power reduced
— Discharge of pus and blood from the ear; pus often pale or milky

Tongue coat: thin
Pulse: floating, rapid

Treatment principle: Expel wind and relieve the exterior, clear heat, and resolve poison.

2. Liver and gall bladder damp-heat

— Inflammation that does not subside
— Headache
— Ear region swollen and painful; eardrum discharges blood; mastoid process mildly painful; outer and middle ear filled with yellow pus
— Stools dry
— May be vomiting and twitching

Tongue coat: greasy, yellow
Tongue body: red
Pulse: wiry, slippery

Treatment principle: Clear heat and bring down damp, resolve poison, reduce swelling, stop pain.

C. Chronic catarrhal

General:

— Tinnitus
— Deafness
— Middle ear full and packed
— Examination shows white distended eardrum.

1. Pathogenic factor remaining

   — Distending and bursting sensation in the middle ear
   — The ear feels blocked. On examination one eardrum
     may be seen to be bleeding slightly or discharging
     clear fluid.
   — May have nose bleed
   — May have nose and throat inflammation
   — May have swollen glands behind the ear and in the
     neck
   — May have recurrent attacks of acute catarrhal otitis

   Pulse: slow or moderate, slippery

   Treatment principle: Move qi and disperse blockage, cir-
   culate blood, and expel the pathogenic factor.

2a. Liver and kidney insufficient

   — Dizziness
   — Sticky fluid on the eardrum
   — May have sore back

   Tongue: tip of tongue red
   Pulse: fine, rapid

   Treatment principle: Support and reinforce liver and kidney; move and regulate the cavities.

2b. Spleen-qi xu and weak

   — Inner ear swollen and bursting
   — Eardrum grey-white in color
   — Patient comparatively lazy and without strength
   — Mouth and lips pale
   — Easily discouraged
   — Poor appetite

   Tongue body: pale
   Pulse: fine, weak

   Treatment principle: Tonify the spleen and bring up jing;
   move the ear cavity, and resolve damp.

Treatment

Main Points

The ear is encircled by the hand shaoyang (sanjiao) channel, and a secondary channel passes through the ear from Fengchi GB-20. Consequently the main points to use are on the hand and foot shaoyang channels:

Fengchi GB-20	To expel wind and regulate the liver and gall bladder
Yifeng SJ-17	To expel wind and benefit the ear
Tinghui GB-2	Local point
Waiguan SJ-5	To expel wind and regulate the sanjiao channel
Zulinqi GB-41	To regulate the liver and gall bladder

Method: Fengchi GB-20 is needled slightly laterally, to direct the sensation to the ear. Yifeng SJ-17 is needled to a depth of 1 cun. Tinghui GB-2 may be needled to a depth of 1½ cun, but in shi conditions it is usually sufficient to needle to a depth of ½ cun. The sensation should radiate to the inner ear and is usually rather painful. Waiguan SJ-5 and Zulinqi GB-41 are needled to a depth of ½ to 1 cun, and the sensation should go upwards along the limb, towards the head.

According to differentiation of syndromes

A. Acute catarrhal

1. Pathogenic wind enters the cavities.

   Provided there are no signs of heat, moxa may be used on Yifeng SJ-17. This will bring quick relief. In addition, add:

   Hegu LI-4   To clear wind

   Prognosis: In babies and young children, one treatment using distal points alone is often enough. The children break out into a sweat, then fall asleep and are cured. Older children may require three treatments (given in one day). If this does not cure the condition, it usually means that it is a different syndrome.

2. Liver and gall bladder oppressed heat

The main points given above are usually sufficient. Alternative points are:

Zhongzhu SJ-3	In place of Waiguan SJ-5
Qiuxu GB-40	In place of Zulinqi GB-41

Prognosis: This condition is common among older children and may take several treatments (three to five) to cure. In cases of very acute pain, give treatment twice or even three times daily. After that, once a day.

B. Acute purulent

1. Pathogenic wind-heat

In addition to the main points, the following points will be of use:

Hegu LI-4	These three points used together
Dazhui Du-14	are very effective in clearing
Quchi LI-11	pathogenic wind-heat.

If there is constipation, a purge should be administered.

Prognosis: One or two treatments are usually sufficient, though it may take more in stubborn cases.

2. Liver and gall bladder damp-heat

In addition to the main points, the following points may be used:

Yinlingquan SP-9	To clear damp-heat
Yanglingquan GB-34	To transform damp in shao yang channel
Zhangmen LIV-13	To transform damp

Method: Four to five points are selected on the affected side. Treat once a day or twice a day in very young children.

Prognosis: This is usually rather slow to change, and there may be no appreciable result until after the third treatment. Usually eight to ten treatments are sufficient.

C. Chronic catarrhal

 1. Pathogenic factor remaining

 In addition to the main points, the following may be of service:

Bailao (extra)	2 cun superior to Dazhui DU-14, one cun lateral to the spine. To clear remaining pathogenic factors.
Ganshu BL-18	To regulate the liver and gall bladder, and move blood and qi.
Pishu BL-20	To regulate the spleen, move blood and qi, and resolve damp.

Method: Needle or moxa may be used on these points.

Prognosis: To clear the body completely of the pathogenic factor may take ten to twenty treatments.

 2a. Liver and kidney insufficient

 Local points are not usually of much service, except in cases of acute pain, and even then their effect is short-term.

 Distal points should be used, e.g.:

Waiguan SJ-5	
Yanglingquan GB-34	These points all have the
Ganshu BL-18	function of tonifying the
Shenshu BL-23	the liver and kidney yin.
Taichong LIV-3	
Taixi KI-3	

Prognosis: This condition is uncommon in children, except after febrile disease, when a few treatments will suffice, provided that the child is eating normally. If the

condition occurs without a history of febrile disease, it
is essential to discover the cause for the yin-xu condition.

2b. Spleen-qi xu and weak

Again, local points are not usually of much service.
Preferable points are:

Waiguan SJ-5	To move qi in the ear
Yanglingquan GB-34	To move qi in the ear
Zusanli ST-36	To tonify the spleen and resolve damp
Sanyinjiao SP-6	To tonify the spleen and resolve damp
Zhongwan REN-12	To tonify the spleen and resolve damp
Hegu LI-4	To tonify the spleen and resolve damp
Pishu BL-20	To tonify the spleen and resolve damp

In babies, Si feng (extra) may be used [located on the
palmar surface, in the transverse creases of the proximal interphalangeal joints of the index, middle, ring,
and little fingers].

Moxa may be used, especially on the abdominal and
back points.

Method: Treat twice or three times a week.

Prognosis: Three to five treatments are usually enough,
provided that the patient can rest.

Notes

1. It is often difficult to distinguish between external
attack of pathogenic wind, and liver and gall bladder
heat conditions, since if there is mental irritation leading to a mild build-up of heat, the child is more susceptible to wind conditions.

2. Repeated treatment with antibiotics can lead to a build-up of damp.

3. In all otitis, the patient should avoid red meat and spicy, fried, and other heating foods. If dampness is present, they should also avoid eggs, cheese, milk, peanuts, and sugar. [Damp conditions are frequently more slow to respond.]

*   *   *

Discharge as a Diagnostic Indicator

Nasal discharge or otorrhea are commonly found in children with otitis media. The color of this discharge often provides useful diagnostic information. Special consideration should be given to the consistency and color of any discharge found. The most common colors are clear, white, yellow, and green.

Discharge	Indication
Clear	Wind-cold, damp
White	Phlegm
Yellow	Heat or bacterial infection
Green	Wind or viral infection

Needle Technique

Needles should be ½ to 1 inch in length and of 32 gauge. They are inserted quickly into the skin, and then manipulated to the required depth to obtain *de qi*. Needle retention is unnecessary in children under 10 years of age,[17] i.e., the needles are quickly withdrawn following *de qi*. A minimum number of needles should be used in children, usually only four to six.[18]

An obstacle that must be overcome when using acupuncture with children is fear of needles. Surprisingly, children do not object to acupuncture to the degree one would expect. More commonly it is the parents who fear needles. If present, these concerns should be dealt with openly before beginning treatment. Acupuncture can be used safely and effectively in children of any age.

Other Forms of Stimulation

Some doctors feel that moxa may be used effectively with children. However, others believe that use of moxa carries a risk of disrupting the San Jiao (triple heater) channel and can have an adverse effect on thermoregulation. I suggest that only the experienced acupuncturist consider using moxa on children, especially in conditions such as otitis media.

It has become popular in China, the United States, and Europe to use various methods of electrical stimulation to treat acupoints. Generally, battery-operated devices that generate a small DC electrical current are either applied to needles inserted into acupoints, or a probe is placed on the point for direct stimulation. I recommend that such devices not be used on children. There are several good reasons for this:

- The levels of current and voltage generated by such devices are high.

- No one is yet certain of the current and voltage thresholds of the body.

- Electrolysis and tissue damage is believed to occur locally when such devices are used.[19]

- Many electrical stimulation devices sold today are subjected to little or no quality control.

Until we more fully understand the direct and indirect effects of this form of stimulation, it is best to use traditional methods.

Si Feng Treatment

According to Martha Benedict, M.A., O.M.D., there is one form of acupuncture treatment that deserves special consideration in the management of otitis media in children. Dr. Benedict has a unique and valuable perspective on otitis media. She has an M.A. in audiology and speech pathology from Stanford

Medical School, and was on the faculty at the University of California Medical Center as a clinician and researcher. After many years of observing the response (and often the lack of response) of thousands of children with otitis media to conventional care, she began her training in Chinese medicine. Her combined experiences in audiology and Chinese medicine have convinced her that most children with otitis media can be effectively treated using acupuncture and Chinese botanical medicine.

One technique used by Dr. Benedict in the management of acute and chronic otitis media is stimulation of the Si Feng points on the palmar surface of the hands. There are twelve Si Feng points. The lower Si Feng is at the metacarpophalangeal joint of the index through little finger. The middle Si Feng is at the proximal interphalangeal joint, and the upper Si Feng at the distal interphalangeal joint. (See figure 18.)

Dr. Benedict treats the middle Si Feng points by applying the technique known as bleeding.* The technique of bleeding acupoints has been used for centuries to manage febrile or inflammatory conditions. This method requires the use of a three-edged needle. When acute or chronic otitis media presents, the needle is used to prick the finger at the locations of the middle Si Feng. This will cause one or two drops of blood to be expressed.

The effects of Si Feng treatment on middle ear inflammation can be impressive. Benedict reports that improvement in the inflammatory state of the middle ear can be observed in as little as ten minutes, often while the child is still in the office. She states that acute otitis often responds fully within 24 hours. The treatment is enhanced when botanicals are used with acupuncture.

---

*Only a trained acupuncturist should attempt this technique.

Figure 18
Location of the Si Feng Points

Botanical Medicine

The clinical use of botanical medicine can have a substantial impact on the underlying syndromes of both acute and chronic otitis media. Children with otitis media who require antibiotic therapy can be assisted by concurrent therapy with botanical medicine. As mentioned above, the use of botanical medicine is enhanced by the simultaneous application of acupuncture and vice versa.

In this section, I present the management of otitis media using Chinese botanical medicine. Admittedly, there are many different traditions of botanical medicine used in the world, all which have intrinsic value. However, the Chinese appear to have developed the most sophisticated and effective method of prescribing for otitis media.

Treatment of Underlying Syndrome

The practitioner of botanical medicine, like the practitioner of acupuncture, relies on a detailed examination of the patient to identify the specific syndrome involved. Once the syndrome is identified, the proper botanical formula is selected based on a few differentiating features. The differentiation of syndromes can be considered the same when using Chinese botanical medicine as when using acupuncture (although the treatment principles may differ somewhat).

Below is a presentation of the Chinese botanical formulas used to manage the various syndromes (described in Chinese medicine) encountered in otitis media.* The format is the same as that presented in the section on acupuncture. For a description of signs and symptoms associated with each syndrome, refer to the section on acupuncture titled "Clinical Manifestations and Differentiation of Syndromes."

---

*This listing of Chinese botanical formulas was compiled by Anastacia White, a professional herbalist. White is a teacher and practitioner of Chinese botanical medicine and lectures throughout the United States.[20]

A. Acute catarrhal

   1. Pathogenic wind enters the cavities

        Formula: Pueraria Combination

        Contains:

Pueraria	*Ma huang*
Peony	*Jujube*
Cinnamon	*Licorice*
Ginger	

        Indications: Used in the early stages when the ear is more stuffed up but without infection.

        Formula: Bupleurum and Schizonepeta

        Contains:

Bupleurum	*Ginger*
Tuhuo	*Hoelen*
Cnidium	*Siler*
Cherry bark	*Licorice*
Platycodon	*Schizonepeta*

        Indications: Used in the early stages when there is slight infection.

   2. Liver and gall bladder oppressed heat

        Formula: Minor Bupleurum

        Contains:

Bupleurum	*Pinellia*
Ginseng	*Licorice*
Ginger	*Jujube*
Scutellaria	

        Indications: Used when the patient has weak stomach and spleen with excessive dampness.

        Formula: Niu Huang Chien Tu Pien

        Contains:

Rhubarb	*Gypsum*
Scutellaria	*Ox gallstone*
Licorice	*Platycodon*
Borneol	

Indications: Used when there are extreme heat symptoms, and the patient does not have a weak spleen.

B. Acute purulent

   1. Wind-heat at the superficial level

      Formula: Schizonepeta and Forsythia

      Contains:

Tang Kuei	*Gardenia*
Scutellaria	*Angelica*
Platycodon	*Peony*
Siler	*Mentha*
Coptis	*Forsythia*
Chih Ko	*Schizonepeta*
Bupleurum	*Rehmannia*
Phellodendron	

   2. Liver and gall bladder damp-heat

      Formula: Gentiana Combination

      Contains:

Gentiana	*Plantago*
Alisma	*Tang Kuei*
Akebia	*Rehmannia*
Gardenia	*Scutellaria*
Licorice	*Bupleurum*

C. Chronic catarrhal

   1. Pathogenic factor remaining

      Formula: Gleditsia Combination

      Contains:

Ginseng	*Atractylodes*
Poria	*Angelica*
Cnidium	*Peony*
Licorice	*Lonicera*
Platycodon	*Tang Kuei*
Gleditsia	*Astragalus*

2a. Liver and kidney insufficient

    Formula: Er Ming Zuo Ci Wan

    Contains:

Rehmannia	*Cornus*
Dioscorea	*Alisma*
Mouton	*Poria*
Bupleurum	*Magnetite Mineral*

2b. Spleen-qi xu and weak

    Formula: Astragalus and Platycodon Combination

    Contains:

Ginseng	*Tang Kuei*
Cnidium	*Licorice*
Cinnamon	*Siler*
Astragalus	*Platycodon*
Angelica	*Magnolia bark*

To further resolve dampness add:

    Formula: Citrus and Pinellia

    Contains:

Citrus	*Licorice*
Ginger	*Poria*
Pinellia	

Symptomatic relief can be provided by using the Superior Sore Throat Powder Spray, which is a Chinese patent formula. The powder is applied by blowing a small amount through a straw into the ear canal. This spray can be used in conjunction with all of the above botanical formulas, with the exception of **Pueraria Combination**.

    Formula: Superior Sore Throat Powder Spray

    Contains:

Coptis	*Ox gallstone*
Borneol	*Mother of pearl*
Licorice	*Indigo powder*
Sophora	

Besides the formulas listed above, a mixture can be prepared for use as eardrops. The combination called "The Three

Yellows" is made from the oils of *Coptis, Phellodendron,* and *Scutellaria*. These are all "cold" herbs, which help to reduce inflammation in the middle ear. A formula known as "The Four Yellows" includes those just mentioned, with the addition of *Astragalus*, which helps eliminate pus. Both are extremely useful in managing the pain associated with otitis media.[21]

Clinical Nutrition

There is no longer any doubt that deficiency of nutrients can lead to disease. There is also no doubt that, under the right circumstances, nutritional therapy can have a substantial impact upon not only amelioration of the symptoms of disease, but the underlying causes as well. As our understanding of nutrition grows, so too do the prospects for treating otitis media with appropriate nutritional intervention.

The nutritional management of otitis media is a somewhat new area. Therefore, rather than listing specific protocols as I've done in prior sections, I will present some relevant research surrounding nutrition as it relates to controlling inflammation and enhancing immune function. This is in the hope that interested persons might expand upon the existing research on nutrition and otitis media.

Nutrition and Inflammation

In chapter 5, I briefly described how fatty acids, vitamins, and minerals affect the formation of both pro-inflammatory and anti-inflammatory prostaglandins. This understanding is important in light of discoveries that inflammatory prostaglandins, leukotrienes, and other arachidonic acid metabolites are found in substantial concentrations in the middle ear fluid of children with otitis media. Among the substances found are PGE2, 6-keto-PGF1 alpha, thromboxane B2, 5-HETE, 15-HETE, leuko triene C4, and leukotriene B4.[22]

Much pharmaceutical research has centered on developing anti-inflammatory drugs that block the formation of inflammatory prostaglandins. These drugs are known as prostaglandin inhibitors. The elder statesmen among these drugs are cortisone and aspirin. The newer generation of PG-inhibitors include indomethacin, acetaminophen, and ibuprofin. As described earlier, besides inhibiting inflammatory prostaglandins, these drugs interfere with the normal production of most other prostaglandins. Thus, there is a great tendency to aggravate the inflammatory response, leading to more chronic health problems.

Nutritional substances, and even botanical medicines, offer an alternative to the use of NSAIDs (Non-Steroidal Anti-Inflammatory Drugs) because they block the enzymes that lead to the production of inflammatory prostaglandins, but do not adversely affect the enzymes needed for conversion of anti-inflammatory prostaglandins. There is evidence that these same nutrients also enhance the formation of the body's natural anti-inflammatory substances.

Using this knowledge, it may be possible to both control the painful symptoms of otitis media and correct the underlying inflammatory imbalance through nutritional intervention.

To understand more clearly the role of nutrients in blocking inflammation, it is necessary to first review the way in which prostaglandins are formed from fatty acids and the various enzymes that are needed for this process.

The Enzymes of Inflammation

Recall that the inflammatory response, as it relates to prostaglandins, begins with the cell membrane. The cell membrane consists of phospholipids that contain a variety of fatty acids. A principal constituent of these phospholipids is arachidonic acid. Arachidonic acid can be present in the cell membrane in large amounts depending upon the level of omega-6 fatty acids in the diet. If omega-3 fatty acids are consumed in large amounts, arachidonic acid is displaced from the phospholipids. (See EPA below.) The enzyme phospholipase A2 catalyzes the liberation of arachidonic acid from the membrane phospholipids, resulting in the creation of free arachidonic acid. This is the first step in the inflammatory pathway known as the arachidonic acid cascade.

Once free arachidonic acid is available, it undergoes further conversion by one of two pathways. Under the action of cyclo-oxygenase, arachidonic acid is converted into thromboxanes or 2-series prostaglandins. Under the action of lipoxygenase, arachidonic acid is converted into derivatives of HPETE (hydroperoxyeicosatetraenoic acid) and leukotrienes. (See figure 19.) Thromboxanes, 2-series prostaglandins, HPETE, and leukotrienes all possess a high degree of inflammation-inducing activity.

Enzymes of the Arachidonic Acid Cascade

1. Phospholipase A2—Causes arachidonic acid stored in the phospholipids of cell membranes to be released as free arachidonic acid. This is the first step toward inflammation via the arachidonic acid cascade.

2. Cyclo-oxygenase—Catalyzes the conversion of free arachidonic acid into prostaglandin E2, prostacyclins, and thromboxanes.

3. Lipoxygenase—Catalyzes the conversion of free arachidonic acid into leukotrienes and HPETEs (and related compounds).

During conditions of excessive or prolonged inflammation, it is often desirable to reduce the substrates available for inflammation. This means balancing the intake of omega-3 and omega-6 fatty acids and in some cases, providing large amounts of certain fatty acids. It is also useful to use nutrients that block enzymes of the inflammatory pathways. Some of these are described below. (See figures 20 and 21.)

Vitamin C. Vitamin C is an important antioxidant nutrient that protects cells from damage by free radicals. Recently, vitamin C was found to be the "premier" antioxidant found in the body.

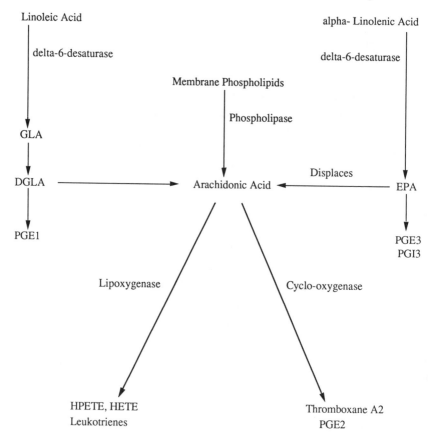

Figure 19

Prostaglandin Synthesis and the Arachidonic Acid Cascade

It was shown to neutralize 100 percent of the free radicals to which it was exposed, while sparing other antioxidants.[23] Vitamin C is necessary for the proper metabolism of drugs and toxic environmental chemicals. It is also necessary for the absorption of iron. The uptake of vitamin C by leukocytes is seriously impaired when traditional anti-inflammatory drugs such as aspirin and cortisone are used. Aspirin taken daily for four days causes the leukocyte levels of ascorbic acid to fall to levels found in scurvy.[24]

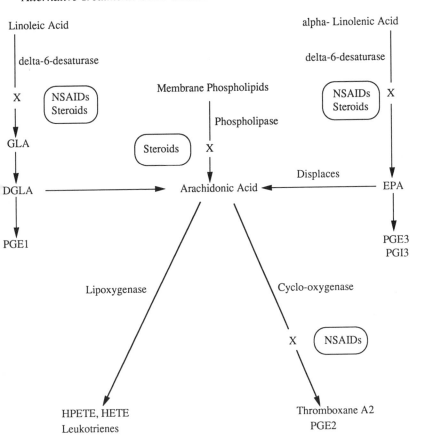

Figure 20

The Effect of Anti-Inflammatory Drugs on Prostaglandins and Arachidonic Acid Metabolites

The "X" indicates where blockage of the pathway occurs. NSAID refers to Non-Steroidal Anti-Inflammatory Drugs. Included in this category are aspirin, acetaminophen, indomethacin, and ibuprofin. Note that NSAIDs favor the formation of lipoxygenase products. These drugs also block the release of the more favorable PGE1 and PGE3 which is undesirable.

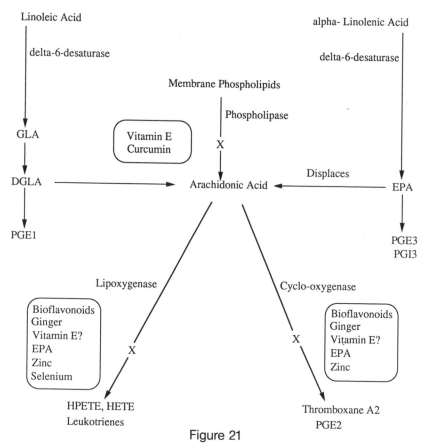

Figure 21

Nutrients That Block the Release of Inflammatory Mediators
The "X" indicates where blockage of the pathway occurs.

Vitamin C does not appear to block the enzymes described above, but it is of vital importance in the detoxification of histamine.[25] Recall that histamine is the chemical responsible for the runny nose, watery eyes, and itchiness associated with hay fever. Histamine also plays an important role in initiating other allergy-related symptoms.

Bioflavonoids. Bioflavonoids are among the few substances that block the action of phospholipase A2, cyclo-oxygenase, and lipoxygenase.[26, 27] Therefore, they interfere with the formation of a whole range of inflammatory prostaglandins. Unlike anti-inflammatory drugs, bioflavonoids do not interfere with the enzymes needed to form PG1, PG3, and other anti-inflammatory prostaglandins. Bioflavonoids are naturally occurring substances commonly found in the same foods as vitamin C. It appears that bioflavonoids enhance the activity of vitamin C.

One example of a bioflavonoid with potent anti-inflammatory action is curcumin, found in the plant *Curcuma longa*, or turmeric. Several studies conducted in the early 1970s show that curcumin has greater anti-inflammatory action than cortisone or NSAIDs. This is, in part, due to its indirect inhibitory effect on phospholipase A2.[28, 29, 30] Curcumin is a potent scavenger of free radicals and may prevent lipid peroxidation more efficiently than beta-carotene and alpha-tocopherol. The substance has thus far been shown to produce no side effects.[31]

Quercitin, another powerful bioflavonoid, is a lipoxygenase inhibitor.[32] The use of quercitin therapeutically prevents the formation of leukotrienes, thereby reducing the symptoms of inflammation.[33] Quercitin also reduces the release of histamine and the IgE-mediated allergic response to food and environmental allergens.[34]

Ginger. Substances derived from the plant *Zingiber officinale* have an inhibitory effect on the enzymes lipoxygenase and cyclo-oxygenase, thus preventing the formation of HPETEs, leukotrienes, thromboxanes, and PG2s.[35] Ginger is among the eight herbs contained in the Japanese formula *Sairei-to*. Recall that this formula was tested for its efficacy in treating otitis media. (See chapter 6.) The authors of this study surmised that part of the action of this formula may be via inhibition of arachidonic acid metabolites.[36]

Vitamin E. Vitamin E is a powerful antioxidant that protects cell membranes against excessive damage from free radicals. It is also an essential factor in preventing blood essential fatty acids from undergoing oxidation. Vitamin E is able to block the enzymes phospholipase A2, lipoxygenase, and cyclo-oxygenase, thereby preventing the release of inflammatory prostaglandins.[37, 38]

Selenium. Selenium is an important part of the anti-oxidant defense system because it is a critical element in the enzyme glutathione peroxidase. This enzyme protects the body's essential fatty acids from destruction. Selenium has a complementary relationship with vitamin E. It potentiates the effects of vitamin E and may compensate to an extent for deficiency of vitamin E.

Zinc. Zinc has many roles to play in the body. It is needed for proper function of delta-6-desaturase and the conversion of fatty acids into prostaglandins. Zinc is also an inhibitor of lipoxygenase and therefore prevents the formation of leukotrienes.[39] The role of zinc deficiency in recurrent otitis media has been described in chapter 5.

GLA (gamma linolenic acid). GLA is a known inhibitor of the inflammatory response. It blocks inflammation by undergoing conversion into the anti-inflammatory PGE1. GLA supplementation may be especially important in children with a history of allergy or eczema. Any child who presents with signs of fatty acid deficiency who also has evidence of delta-6-desaturase inhibition (based on a history of exposure to d-6-d inhibitors) may require supplementation with GLA in addition to linoleic acid. The effective dose in children has been shown to be one capsule per day per year of age up to a maximum of six capsules. Some children who do not respond at this dose may require substantially more.[40]

EPA (eicosapentaenoic acid). EPA is incorporated into the membranes of cells, where it displaces arachidonic acid. This reduces the amount of arachidonic acid (or substrate) available for the inflammatory response. EPA is converted into PGE3, exerting an inhibitory effect on the enzymes cylco-oxygenase and lipoxygenase. EPA also appears to potentiate the effect of the other anti-inflammatory prostaglandin, PGE1.[41] Any child who presents with signs of fatty acid deficiency who also has evidence of delta-6-desaturase inhibition (based on a history of exposure to d-6-d inhibitors) may require supplementation with EPA in addition to linolenic acid.

Beta-Carotene. Beta-carotene, also known as pro-vitamin A, has at least two important functions. Beta-carotene itself is an important anti-oxidant. Clearly, the anti-oxidants do not work alone, but in concert with one another. Therefore, it is important that all anti-oxidants be present in adequate amounts. Beta-carotene is also important because a percentage of dietary beta-carotene undergoes conversion to vitamin A. The importance of vitamin A in otitis media has already been discussed. Both vitamin A and beta-carotene should be present in the diet since the conversion of beta-carotene to vitamin A is believed by some to be insufficient to supply all the vitamin A needs.

A Consideration: Fetal Alcohol Syndrome

In chapter 5, I described the many factors that, individually or in concert, interfere with the proper conversion of fatty acids by blocking the enzyme delta-6-desaturase. Dr. David Horrobin has shown that infants have a poorly developed d-6-d system. He has also shown that intake of alcohol causes the enzyme to be blocked. Since roughly 10 percent of all calories consumed by people in North America are in the form of alcohol,[42] an important question is raised regarding Fetal Alcohol Syndrome (FAS).

FAS is a condition that affects children born to mothers who have consumed alcohol during the gestational period. The understanding of this syndrome today relates primarily to behavior and motor problems, and to growth irregularities. FAS was originally believed to affect children of alcoholic mothers. However, we now know that even moderate alcohol consumption during pregnancy (as few as one or two drinks) can lead to varying degrees of FAS.

Here is the connection. Alcohol adversely affects the enzyme delta-6-desaturase and can produce significant adverse changes in the children of mothers who consume alcohol just before conception or during pregnancy. Given this, it is conceivable that one of the manifestations of FAS might be impaired fatty acid metabolism due to poorly functioning enzymes. Impaired fatty acid metabolism would, in part, explain some of the behavioral and motor problems of FAS children, since the nervous system is highly dependent upon the proper metabolism of fats. (Obviously, there are numerous additional factors that go beyond this.)

FAS is now as prevalent as Down syndrome (between one in 500 and one in 1,000 births).[43, 44] Children with FAS have an incidence of otitis media equivalent to children with Down syndrome and cleft palate.[45] In addition, there may be a substantial population of children who do not have classic signs of FAS, yet have been adversely affected by mild or moderate consumption of alcohol by the mother. These children would not be recognized as having FAS. Yet there may be sufficient enzyme impairment to significantly disrupt their normal fatty acid metabolism. This would result in a condition favoring inflammation. Theoretically, these children would be at greater risk to inflammatory conditions such as otitis media.

Children with defective d-6-d enzymes would not be expected to respond to any conventional therapy (such as antibiotics or surgery) because they would suffer from an inherent inability to combat inflammation. In such children, even supplementation with linoleic acid, linolenic acid, and co-factors would fail because the enzymes would be unable to convert the fatty acids into PGE1, PGE3, and related compounds. Most likely, substantial amounts GLA, EPA, and co-factors would be required. This would by-pass the step where d-6-d is required and provide the needed raw material to manufacture

PG1 and PG3.* (See figure 19.) Presently this idea is only a hypothesis. It, however, deserves consideration since up to 93 percent of children with FAS suffer from recurrent otitis media.[46]

Nutrition and Immune Function

Nutrition is rapidly being shown to play a crucial role in many aspects of immune function. There are solid indications that nutritional supplementation can have a direct and significant effect on the outcome of infection. Below is a discussion of nutrients known to play a role in immune function.

Zinc. Zinc is perhaps the most extensively researched nutrient with regard to immune function. Deficiency adversely affects T and B-cell function, thymic size, and resistance to viruses, bacteria, and parasites. Zinc deficiency can impair both the primary and secondary immune response.[47, 48, 49, 50, 51, 52] It has been estimated that roughly three-fourths of the American population are zinc-deficient.[53]

Copper. Copper deficiency has been associated with decreased immune competence and increased incidence of infection.[54] Excessive zinc intake can lead to copper deficiency. Excessive zinc levels sometimes occur in individuals who are taking zinc as a supplement. Copper excess has also been linked to immune impairment. When copper is present in excessive amounts, it exerts an antagonistic effect on zinc, leading to zinc deficiency.

Selenium. Deficiency of selenium results in diminished resistance to microbial and viral infections, neutrophil function,

---

*This additional need for GLA and EPA should also be considered in diabetic children who suffer from recurrent otitis media. Juvenile onset diabetes is complex and should be managed carefully. Any nutritional changes should only be undertaken after consultation with a doctor.

antibody production, and reduced ability of T-cells and natural killer cells to destroy pathogens. Supplementation with selenium has been shown to reverse these processes. This trace element has been said to ". . . affect all components of the immune system."[55]

Germanium. Germanium is an immune-potentiating trace element when used therapeutically. Germanium is known to stimulate interferon production and is considered an immune-regulator. It is believed to have anti-oxidant properties as well.[56]

Vitamin C. The effects of vitamin C on immune function have been widely publicized. Vitamin C appears to stimulate interferon production, enhance T-lymphocyte function, enhance antibody formation, and reduce the adverse effects of environmental chemicals. Vitamin C plays an important role in white cell phagocytosis.[57] Esterified L-ascorbic acid appears to be the most effective for use in acute infections when rapid uptake is required. Recent evidence suggests that ingestion of esterified ascorbic acid results in twice the blood levels and four times the tissue levels when compared to ascorbate and citrate forms. Esterified forms are also excreted less rapidly, which is desirable when lasting action is needed.[58]

Bioflavonoids. The bioflavonoid quercitin has been shown to inhibit the replication of several viruses including herpes simplex type 1, polio virus type 1, parainfluenzal virus type 3, and respiratory syncytial virus.[59, 60]

Vitamin E. Vitamin E exerts an effect on the immune system through its role as an antioxidant. It also affects immune function by regulating the formation of prostaglandins. Vitamin E exerts a protective effect on vitamin A. Also, when vitamin E is deficient, vitamin A absorption is impaired.[61, 62] Excessive vitamin E intake has an immunosuppressive effect.[63]

Pyridoxine. Pyridoxine deficiency results in depressed humoral and cell-mediated immunity and inhibition of the antibody response.[64] Anecdotal reports have shown an increased incidence of otitis media associated with pyridoxine deficiency. Supplementation of pyridoxine should not be undertaken without adequate B-vitamins, since conversion of pyridoxine to the active pyridoxal-5-phosphate requires riboflavin and may require other nutrients.

Beta-carotene. Beta-carotene is one of the most potent free-radical scavengers yet discovered. It is of major importance in protecting the cellular lining of the lungs and respiratory tract. There is evidence that it plays a similar role in the lining of the eustachian tube and tympanic cavity. Modest doses appear to stimulate the immune response.[65]

Vitamin A. Vitamin A deficiency results in thymic and splenic atrophy, and a reduction in the numbers of circulating leukocytes and lymphocytes.[66] Supplementation may reverse these effects. Excessive vitamin A (retinol or retinoic acid) can be immunosuppressive.[67] Whenever vitamin A is given therapeutically, beta-carotene should also be given. Beta-carotene appears to prevent the macrophage inhibition that can occur with vitamin A supplementation.

Fat. Excessive fat intake or elevated blood fats (cholesterol or triglycerides) tend to decrease resistance to bacterial and viral infections.[68] Linoleic acid, linolenic acid, and eicosapentaenoic acid all have been shown to have anti-bacterial, anti-fungal, and anti-viral activity.[69]

Pantothenic acid. Pantothenic acid is a water-soluble vitamin that is greatly affected by stress and illness. During these times, the adrenal glands require large amounts of pantothenic acid. When pantothenic acid is deficient, the adrenal glands begin to atrophy.[70] During deficiency there is an increased susceptibility to infection, decrease in gamma globulin concentrations, impaired antigenic response, and poor viral and bacterial defenses.[71, 72]

Thymus tissue. Within the past ten years, substantial documentation has confirmed the value of raw bovine thymus tissue supplementation in cases of recurrent infections and decreased immunocompetence. Ingestion of oral thymus tissue can enhance T and B lymphocyte formation, increase T helper levels and activity, and balance T helper/suppressor ratios.[73, 74, 75] Bovine thymus tissue is known to contain thymosin, serum thymic factor, thymopoieten, and other biologically active substances.[76] Thymus tissue appears to be effective in the treatment of acute and chronic infections. Only thymus tissue that has been defatted or azeotrophically processed should be used because of the possibility of contamination by bovine slow viruses.[77]

*   *   *

There is yet no standard or accepted protocol for the nutritional management of otitis media. This is because our understanding of nutrition as it relates to inflammation/infection is only now emerging. The second reason is that the possibility of a nutritional role in otitis media has gained little attention within the medical community. While deficiency of certain nutrients seem to be common in recurrent otitis media, there are a host of other nutritional factors that may be important in a given child. Therefore, this final chapter is intended as a starting point.

The nutritional recommendations given in chapter 6 are based on a general knowledge of nutrition and immunity, and nutrition and inflammation. It is a basic approach that may be helpful for some children. The practitioner who is confronted with a child with recurrent otitis media must consider the full range of diagnostic possibilities—both nutritional and otherwise. Any therapeutic nutritional program that is undertaken should be done concurrently with an elimination of anti-nutrients such as trans fatty acids, heavy metals, sugar, and others.

Epilogue

Otitis media affects children at all points on the socioeconomic spectrum. At one extreme, nearly one-fifth of all children under the age of six live at or below the poverty level. These children often live in highly stressful environments where hygiene is less than optimal and proper nutrition is lacking. Among these children, the incidence of recurrent otitis media is high. The impact on their mental and emotional development can be severe, often lasting into adulthood. The physical and emotional needs of these children must be met through an influx of economic and human resources. Resources to provide adequate nutrition must be a top priority.

At the other end of the spectrum lie children growing up in more affluent environments. At first glance, one might think these children are at lower risk to developing otitis media and learning problems than their less fortunate cohorts. However, affluent children (and children from middle class families) are commonly victims of "overconsumptive undernutrition" as described by Dr. Jeffrey Bland. This a condition in which caloric intake is more than adequte, but the calories are not accompanied by the nutrients necessary for optimal health. Affluent families have sufficient resources to provide good nutrition for their children, but frequently lack the knowledge, initiative, or will power to implement the needed changes.

The medical profession has for too long ignored the critical importance of diet and nutrition in diseases of children. Food allergy and sensitivity is vastly underrated by many family physicians. In most doctors, knowledge of the signs of nutritional deficiency is lacking. Otolaryngologists commonly focus their efforts upon surgery. This is why we must look to holistic doctors of all backgrounds for guidance. Holistic doctors view diet, lifestyle, environment, emotions, and spirituality as cornerstones of good health. They are more inclined to treat the child as opposed to treating the disease. They are less inclined to use drugs and surgery as their first choice in treating illness. It is these individuals who have the viewpoint that is so urgently needed as we tackle the problem of childhbood otitis media.

Parents and doctors must recognize that no system of medicine can claim total success in the treatment of disease. In the United States, we spend almost four times more money on health care than any other industrialized nation. In spite of this, our infant mortality rate is among the worst in the industrialized world. Our life expectancy is less than one would expect considering the resources expended on health care. This reflects the odd marriage of a medicine which is highly reliant upon technology, yet often fails to attend to basic needs. What is required to solve many of our current health problems is an open dialolgue between those in allopathic medicine and those in holistic medicine. We must establish a complementary relationship between the two sciences. In areas where allopathic medicine excels, it should be the method of choice. In areas where holistic medicine excels, holistic medicine should be employed. In some instances, concurrent use may be best. Failure to recognize the benefits of each system potentially deprives us of the care needed to adequately solve our health problems.

Had allopathic doctors not listened to the wisdom of Chinese botanical medicine, the World Health Organization might never have learned of the plant *Artemisia annua*—recently found to be one of the most effective treatments for *Giardia* yet discovered. This plant has been used in the treatment of febrile illness and parasitic infection for centuries. How many other pearls of medical wisdom lie buried in the archives of ancient and traditional medicine? Are doctors willing to ignore potentially beneficial treatments for otitis media because of differing philosophies?

My primary goal in writing this book is to educate the public. My second, but equally important goal is to open a dialogue and perhaps bridge the gap between two schools of thought. I have pointed out weaknesses in the current treatment of otitis media and have offered alternatives. While some doctors may object to the very idea that holistic methods have merit in the care of otitis media, I am certain there are many doctors who are openly looking for solutions irrespective of their philosophical beliefs.

To stem the rising tide of ear infections in children, we must enlist the help of all people, including parents, doctors, day care providers, educators, and public health officials. As a society, we must redefine our lifestyles and change our eating habits. Parents must demand that their doctors be knowledgeable in the intricacies of nutritional medicine. Parents must no longer surrender responsibility for the health of their children to doctors, but instead must engage in a partnership with their doctors.

Doctors in holistic medicine must educate the public about the benefits of their approach. Moreover, they must continue to conduct quality research and provide documentation that will withstand scientific scrutiny. Allopathic doctors must take a more cautious approach to the use of antibiotics and tubes. Most importantly, allopathic and holistic doctors must engage in a cooperative effort so that their collective insights might bring about the most expedient and effective solutions to our number one pediatric health problem.

Appendix

Resources

Listed below are companies that sell various health-related products. This list is not an endorsement of any company or product. It is for informational purposes only. Note that some companies market only to health care professionals and prefer not to respond to inquiries from the public. These are indicated with an asterisk.

Nutritional Products

Metagenics, Inc.*
23180 Del Lago
Laguna Hills, CA 92653
714-855-1718

Nutrition Dynamics*
5410 Highway 12
Maple Plain, MN 55359
800-444-9998

NutriCology, Inc.
400 Preda Street
San Leandro, CA 94577
800-545-9960

Spectrum Naturals
133 Copeland Street
Petaluma, CA 94952
707-778-8900

Homeopathic Medicine

Biological Homeopathic
  Industries*
11600 Cochiti S. E.
Albuquerque, NM 87123
800-621-7644

Boiron-Bornemann
1208 Amosland Road
Norwood, PA 19074
800-258-8823

Boericke & Tafel, Inc.
2381 Circadian Way
Santa Rosa, CA 95407
800-876-9505

Homeopathic Educational
  Services
2124 Kittredge Avenue
Berkeley, CA 94704
415-649-0294 (inquiries)
800-359-9051 (orders)

Standard Homeopathic Co.
210 W. 131st Street
Los Angeles, CA 90061
800-624-9659

Botanical Medicine

K'an Herb Company*
2425 Porter Street, Suite 18
Soquel, CA 95073
800-543-5233

I.T.M.*
2442 S. E. Sherman
Portland, OR 97214
800-544-7504

Brion Herb Corporation*
12020 B. Centralia Rd.
Hawaiian Gardens, CA 90716
800-333-HERB

McZand Herbal, Inc.*
P.O. Box 5312
Santa Monica, CA 90405
213-392-8404

Acupuncture

OMS Medical Supplies, Inc.*
1950 Washington Street
Braintree, MA 02184
800-323-1839

Redwing Book Company
44 Linden Street
Brookline, MA 02146
800-873-3946

Organizations

American Academy of
  Environmental Medicine
P.O. Box 16106
Denver, CO 80216

Candida Research Information
  Foundation
P.O. Box 2719
Castro Valley, CA 94546
(415) 582-2179

Human Ecology Action League
  (HEAL)
P.O. Box 66637
Chicago, IL 60666
(312) 665-6575

International Health Foundation
William Crook, M.D.
800-372-7665

American Holistic Medical
  Association
2727 Fairview Avenue E.
Seattle, WA 98102
(206) 322-6842

International College of
  Applied Kinesiology
10540 Marty, Suite 240
Shawnee Mission, KS 66212
(913) 648-2828

American Chiropractic
  Association
1701 Clarendon Boulevard.
Arlington, VA 22209

American Osteopathic
  Association
212 East Ohio Street
Chicago, IL 60611
(312) 280-5800

National Resources Defense
  Council
800-648-NRDC

National Center for Homeopathy
1500 Massachusetts Avenue N.W.
Washington, DC 20005
(202) 223-6182

American Institute of
  Homeopathy
1500 Massachusetts Avenue N.W.
Washington, DC 20005

International Foundation for
  Homeopathy
2366 Eastlake Avenue E. #301
Seattle, WA 98102

British Homeopathic Association
27A Devonshire Street
London, W1N 1RJ, England

Foundation for Homeopathic
  Education & Research
5916 Chabot Crest
Oakland, CA 94618
(415) 649-8930

National Commission for the
  Certification of Acupuncturists
1424 16th Street N.W.
Suite 501
Washington, DC 20036
(202) 323-1404

American Academy of
  Acupuncture and Oriental
  Medicine
1424 16th Street N.W.
Suite 501
Washington, DC 20036
(202) 265-2287

Institute for Traditional Medicine
2017 S.E. Hawthorne
Portland, OR 97214
800-544-7504

Suggested Reading

The books marked with an asterisk are those that would be of interest primarily to health professionals. All others would be of interest to the general reader.

General

Lappé, M.; *When Antibiotics Fail: Restoring the Ecology of the Body*, North Atlantic Books, Berkeley, California, 1986.

Mendelsohn, R.S.; *How to Raise a Healthy Child in Spite of Your Doctor*, Contemporary Books, Chicago, Illinois, 1984.

Allergy

Roberts, S.; *The EI Syndrome: Rx for Environmental Illness*, Prestige Publishers, New York, 1989.

Crook, W.; *Are You Allergic*, Professional Books, Jackson, Tennessee, 1974.

Randolph, T.; *An Alternative Approach to Allergies*, Lippincott & Crowell, New York, 1980.

Jones, M.; *The Allergy Self-Help Cookbook*, Rodale Press, Inc., Emmaus, Pennsylvania, 1984.

Homeopathic Medicine

Ullman, D., *Homeopathy: Medicine for the 21st Century*, North Atlantic Books, Berkeley, California, 1988.

Vithoulkas, G.; *The Science of Homeopathy*, Grove Press, New York, 1980.*

Santwani, M.; *Common Ailments of Children and Their Homeopathic Management*, Jain Publishing Company, New Dehli, 110055, 1983.

Cummings, S.; Ullman, D.; *Everybody's Guide to Homeopathic Medicines*, Jeremy P. Tarcher, Los Angeles, 1984.

Herscu, P.; *The Homeopathic Treatment of Children: Pediatric Constitutional Types*, North Atlantic Books, Berkeley, California, 1990.*

Kent, J.T.; *Repertory of Homeopathic Materia Medica*, Jain Publishing Company, New Dehli, 110055.*

Wheeler, C.E.; Kenyon, J.D.; *An Introduction to the Principles and Practice of Homeopathy*, Daniel Company, London, 1980.

Boericke, W.; *Pocket Manual of Materia Medical with Repertory*, Indian Books & Periodical Syndicate, New Dehli, 110055.*

Coulter. H.; *Homeopathic Science and Modern Medicine*, North Atlantic Books, Berkeley, California, 1980.

Messer, S.; *Otitis Media in Children*, Homeopathic Educational Services, Berkeley, California, 1986 (audio tape).*

Chinese Medicine

Bensky; Gamble; *Chinese Herbal Medicine Materia Medica*, Eastland Press, Seattle, Washington, 1986.*

Hsu, H.Y.; Hsu, C.S.; *Commonly Used Chinese Herbal Formulas*, Oriental Healing Arts Institute, Los Angeles, California, 1980.*

Yeung, H.; *Handbook of Chinese Herbs and Formulas*, Institute of Chinese Medicine, Los Angeles, California, 1983.*

Dharmananda, S.; *Foundations of Chinese Herb Prescribing*, The Institute for Traditional Medicine, Portland, Oregon, 1989.*

Tierra, M.; *Planetary Herbology*, Lotus Light, Wilmot, Wisconsin, 1988.*

Pang, T.Y.; *Chinese Herbal: An Introduction*, Tai Chi School of Philosophy and Art, East Sound, Washington, 1982.*

Fratkin, J.; *Chinese Herbal Patent Forumulas*, The Institute for Traditional Medicine, Portland, Oregon, 1986.*

Flaws, B.; Wolfe, H.L.; *Prince Wen Hui's Cook: Chinese Dietary Therapy*, Paradigm Publications, Brookline, Massachusetts, 1983.

Flaws, B.; *Turtle Tail and Other Tender Mercies: Traditional Chinese Pediatrics*, Blue Poppy Press, Boulder, Colorado, 1985.*

Scott, J.; *The Treatment of Children by Acupuncture*, The Journal of Chinese Medicine, Sussex, England, 1986.*

Kaptchuck, T.; *The Web That Has No Weaver*, Congdon & Weed, New York, 1983.*

Ross, J.; *Zang Fu: The Organ Systems of Chines Medicine*, second edition, Churchill Livingstone, New York, 1985.*

Porkert, M.; Ullman, C.; *Chinese Medicine: It's History, Philosophy & Practice, & Why it May One Day Dominate the Medicine of the West*, William Morrow and Company, 1988.

Matsumoto, K.; Birch, S.; *Five Elements and Ten Stems*, Paradigm Publications, Brookline, Massachusetts, 1983.*

Firebra, P.; et al; *Acupuncture: The Illustrated Guide*, Harmony Books, New York, 1988.

Kenyon, J.; *Acupressure Techniques: A Self-Help Guide*, Healing Arts Press, Rochester, Vermont, 1988.

Chiropractic/Osteopathy

Maitland, G.D.; *Vertebral Manipulation*, fifth edition, Butterworths, London, 1986.*

Buerger, A.A.; Greenman, P.E.; *Empirical Approaches to the Validation of Spinal Manipulation*, Charles C. Thomas, Springfield, Illinois, 1985.*

Dryburgh, R.A.; *So You're Thinking of Going to a Chiropractor*, Keats Publishing, Inc., New Canaan, Connecticut, 1984.

Chiropractic State of the Art 1987-1988, American Chiropractic Association, Arlington, Virginia, 1988.

Kelner, M.; Hall, O.; Coulter, I.;*"Chiropractors: Do They Help?"* Fitzhenry and Whiteside, Toronto, Canada, 1980.

Nutrition

Erasmus, U.; *Fats and Oils: The Complete Guide to Fats and Oils in Health and Nutrition*, Alive Press, Vancouver, Canada, 1986.

Rudin, D.O.; Felix, C.; *The Omega-3 Phenomenon*, Avon Books, New York, 1987.

Galland, L.; *Superimmunity for Kids*, E.P. Dutton, New York, 1988.

Bland, J.S.; et al.; *The 1984-85 Yearbook of Nutritional Medicine*, Keats Publishing, New Canaan, Connecticut, 1985.*

Werbach, M.; *Nutritional Influences on Illness: A Sourcebook of Clinical Research*, Third Line Press, Tarzana, California, 1988.*

Smith, L.H.; *Feed Your Kids Right*, Dell Publishing Co., Inc., New York, 1979.

Grand, R.J.; et al; *Pediatric Nutrition: Theory and Practice*, Butterworths, Boston, 1987.*

Shills, M.E.; Young, V.R.; *Modern Nutrition in Health and Disease*, Lea & Febiger, Philadelphia, 1988.*

Nutrition Reviews' Present Knowledge in Nutrition, fifth edition, The Nutrition Foundation, Inc., Washington, D.C., 1984.*

*   *   *

We are currently gathering information on the holistic management of otitis media. If you have clinical data, research reports, or detailed case studies that you think would help improve our understanding of this condition please send them to:

>Otitis Media Research
>Brookview Health Sciences
>P.O. Box 452
>Anoka, MN 55303

References

Introduction

1. Diamant, M.; Diamant, B.; "Abuse and Timing of Use of Antibiotics in Acute Otitis Media," *Arch. Otolaryngol.* 100:226-232, 1974.

2. Van Buchem, F.L.; "Therapy of Acute Otitis Media: Myringotomy, Antibiotics, or Neither? A Double-Blind Study in Children," *Lancet* 883, Oct. 24, 1981.

3. Chaput de Saintonge, D.M.; Levine, D.F.; et al.; "Trial of Three-Day and Ten-Day Courses of Amoxycillin in Otitis Media," *Br. Med. J.* Vol. 284, Apr. 10, 1982.

4. Brown, M.J.; Richards, S.H.; Ambegaoker, A.G.; "Grommets and Glue Ear: A Five-Year Follow-Up of a Controlled Trial," *J. Roy. Soc. Med.* Vol. 71:353-356, 1978.

5. Pang, L.Q.; "The Importance of Allergy in Otolaryngology," *Clinical Ecology,* Dickey, L. (Ed.), Charles Thomas, Springfield, Illinois, p. 633, 1976.

6. Skoner, D.P.; Stillwagon, P.K.; et al.; "Inflammatory Mediators in Chronic Otitis Media with Effusion," *Arch. Otolaryngol. Head Neck Surg.* Vol. 114, 1131-1133, Oct., 1988.

7. Bondestam, M.; Foucard, T.; Gebre-Medhin, M.; "Subclinical Trace Element Deficiency in Children with Undue Susceptibility to Infections," *Act. Paed. Sc.* 74:515-520, 1985.

Chapter 1 The Scope of the Problem

1. Eisenberg, L.; "Preventive Pediatrics: The Promise and the Peril," *Pediatrics* Vol. 80, No. 3, pp. 415-416, 1987.

2. Asman, B.J.; Fireman, P.; "The Role of Allergies in the Development of Otitis Media with Effusion," *Intl. Ped.* Vol 3, No. 3, pp. 231-233, July-Sept., 1988.

3. Teele, D.W.; Klein, J.O.; Rosner, B.A.; "Epidemiology of Otitis Media in Children," *Ann-Otol-Rhinol-Laryngol* [Suppl.] 89(3 Pt 2 Suppl. 68), pp. 5-6, May-June, 1980.

17. Schwartz, D.M.; Schwartz, R.H.; "Acoustic Impedance and Otoscopic Findings in Young Children with Down's Syndrome," *Arch. Otoloaryngol.* 104:652, 1978.

18. Backman, A.; Bjorksten, F.; et al.; "Do Infections in Infancy Affect Sensitization to Airborne Allergens and Development of Atopic Disease? A Retrospective Study of Seven-Year-Old Children," *Allergy* 39(4), pp. 309-15, May, 1984.

19. Draper, W.L.; "Secretory Otitis Media," *Clinical Ecology*, Dickey, L. (Ed.), Charles Thomas, Springfield, Illinois, pp. 176-178, 1976.

20. Bondestam, M.; Foucard, T.; Gebre-Medhin, M.; "Subclinical Trace Element Deficiency in Children with Undue Susceptibility to Infections," *Act. Paed. Sc.* 74:515-520, 1985.

21. "Report of a Survey by the Medical Research Council's Working-party for Research in General Practice: Acute Otitis Media in General Practice," *Lancet* 2:510, 1957.

22. Gutmann, G.; "Das Atlas-Blockierungs-Syndrome des Sauglings und des Kleinkindes," *Manuelle Med.* 25:5-10, 1987.

23. Howie, V.M.; Ploussard, J.H.; Sloyer, J.; "The 'Otitis-Prone' Condition," *Am. J. Dis. Child.* 129:676-8, 1975.

24. Roberts, J.E.; Burchinal, M.R.; et al.; "Otitis Media in Early Childhood and Cognitive, Academic, and Classroom Performance of the School-Aged Child," *Pediatrics* Vol. 83, No. 4, Apr., 1989.

25. Paradise, J.L.; "Management of Secretory Otitis Media: State of the Art," *Adv. Oto-Rhino-Laryng.* Vol. 40, p. 103, 1988.

26. Karma, P.; et al.; "Finnish Approach to the Treatment of Acute Otitis Media: Report of the Finnish Consensus Conference," *Ann. Otol. Rhinol. Laryngol.* 97: 1988.

27. Lildholt, T.; Kortholm, B.; "Beclomethasone Nasal Spray in the Treatment of Middle Ear Effusion: A Double-blind Study," *Int. J. Pediat. Otorhinolar.* 4:133-137, 1982.

28. Jung, T.T.K.; "Arachidonic Acid Metabolites in Otitis Media Pathogenesis," *Ann. Otol. Rhinol. Laryngol.* 97:1988.

29. Doran, T.F.; DeAngelis, C.; Baumgardner, R.A.; Mellitis, E.D.; "Acetaminophen: More Harm Than Good for Chickenpox?" *J. Pediatrics* 114(6):1045-8, 1989.

30. Cantekin, E.I.; Mandel, E.M.; Bluestone, C.D.; Rockette, H.E.; Paradise, J.L.; et al.; "Lack of Efficacy of a Decongestant-Antihistamine Combination for Otitis Media with Effusion ('secretory otitis media') in Children. Results of a Double-blind, Randomized Trial," *New Engl. J. Med..* 308:297-301, 1983.

31. Southcott, R.V.; *Med. J. Aust.* ii, 281, 1953.

32. Chaitow, L.; *Vaccination and Immunization: Dangers, Delusions, and Alternatives*, C.W. Daniel Company Limited, England, 1987.

33. Sade, J.; *Secretory Otitis Media and Its Sequelae.* Churchill Livingstone, Inc., 1979.

34. Fiellau-Nikolajsen, M.; "Adenoidectomy for Eustachian Tube Dysfunction: Long-term Results from a Randomized Controlled Trial," *Acta. Otolaryngol.* Suppl., 386:129, 1982.

35. Widemar, L.; "The Effect of Adenoidectomy on Secretory Otitis Media," *Acta. Otolaryngol.* Suppl., 386:132, 1983.

36. Elverland, H.H.; "Adenoidectomy and Secretory Otitis Media," *Acta. Otolaryngol.* Suppl., 386:134, 1983.

37. Mendelsohn, R.S.; "Ear Infections . . . Tubes in Ears . . . Ear Noises," *The People's Doctor* Vol. 5, No. 5, 1985.

38. Bluestone, C.D.; et al.; "Controversies in Antimicrobial Agents for Otitis Media," *Ann. Otol. Rhinol. Laryngol.* Suppl., 1988.

39. Roddey, O.F.; Earle, R.; Haggerty, R.; "Myringotomy in Acute Otitis Media: A Controlled Study," *J.A.M.A.* 197:849, 1966.

40. Paradise, J.L.; "Management of Secretory Otitis Media: State of the Art," *Adv. Oto-Rhino-Laryng.* Vol. 40, pp. 99-109, 1988.

41. Samuels, M.; Samuels, N.; *The Well Baby Book*, Summit Books, N.Y., pp. 270-272, 1979.

42. Juselius, H.; Kaltiokallio, K.; "Complications of Acute and Chronic Otitis Media in the Antibiotic Era," *Acta. Otolaryngol.* (Stockh) 74:445, 1972.

43. Shaffer, H.L.; "Acute Masoiditis and Cholesteatoma," *Otolaryngology* 86:394, 1978.

44. Pfaltz, C.R.; "Complications of Acute Otitis Media in Children," *Adv. Oto-Rhino-Laryng.* Vol. 40, pp. 70-80, 1988.

45. Paparella, M.M.; Goycoolea, M.; et al.; "Silent Otitis Media: Clinical Applications," *Laryngoscope* 96:978-985, Sept. 1986.

46. Froom, J.; "Clinical Review: Otitis Media," *J. Fam. Pract.* Vol. 15, No. 4:743-770, 1982.

Chapter 2 Antibiotics: Sensible Use or Abuse?

1. Galland, L.; Buchman, D.D.; *SuperImmunity for Kids*, E.P. Dutton, New York, p. 201, 1988.

2. Lildholdt, T.; "Unilateral Grommet Insertion and Adenoidectomy in Bilateral Secretory Otitis Media: Preliminary Report of the Results in 91 Children," *Clin. Otolaryngol.* 4:87-93, 1979.

3. Fabricious, H.F.; "Hearing Investigation of School Children in North Trondelay County," *J. Oslo City Hospital* 18:3, 1968.

4. "Pediatric Antibiotic Use Soars (As Adult Prescriptions Slide)," *Medical World News* November 9, 1987.

5. Nelson, W.; Conference on Antimicrobial Agents and Chemotherapy, FDA Report, New York, 1987.

6. "Pediatric Antibiotic Use Soars (As Adult Prescriptions Slide)," *Medical World News* November 9, 1987.

7. Lappé, M.; *When Antibiotics Fail: Restoring the Ecology of the Body*, North Atlantic Books, Berkeley, California, 1986.

8. Schwartz, R.; Rodriguez, W.; Khan, W.; Ross, S.; "The Increasing Incidence of Ampicillin-Resistant *Haemophilus influenzae* : A Cause of Otitis Media," *J.A.M.A.* Vol. 239, No. 4, Jan. 23, 1978.

9. Georghiou, G.P., "The Magnitude of the Resistance Problem," in NRC, Board of Agriculture, Pesticide Resistance: Strategies and Tactics for Management, National Academy Press, Washington, D.C., 1986.

10. *Drug Information,* American Hospital Formulary Service, American Society of Hospital Pharmacists, Inc., Bethesda, MD, p. 218, 1986.

11. Welch, H.G.; "Antibiotic Resistance: A New Kind of Epidemic," *Postgraduate Medicine* Vol. 76, No. 6, Nov. 1, 1984.

12. Crossley, K.; et al.; "An Outbreak of Infections Caused by Strains of S. aureus Resistant to Methicillin and Aminoglycosides," *J. Infect. Dis.* 139:273-87, 1979.

13. Belsheim, J.A.; Gnarpe, G.H.; "Antibiotics and Granulocytes; Direct and Indirect Effects on Granulocyte Chemotaxis," *Acta. Path. Mocrobiol. Scand.* Sect C, 89:217:221, 1981.

14. Gillon, J.; "Protozoan Infections of the GI Tract," *Quart. J. Med.* 52:29-39, 1984.

15. Pickering, L.K.; Woodward, W.E.; "Diarrhea in Day Care Centers," *Ped. Infect. Dis. J.* Vol. 1, No. 1, pp. 47-51, 1982.

16. Nussenzweigh, R.S.; "Parasitic Disease as a Cause of Immunosuppression," *New Engl. J. Med.* Feb. 18, 1982.

17. Burdon, D.W.; "Treatment of Pseudomembranous Colitis and Antibotic-Associated Diarrhea," *J. Antimicr. Chemoth.* 14 Suppl. D, pp. 103-109, 1984.

18. Helstrom, P.B.; Balish, E.; "Effect of Oral Tetracycline, the Microbial Flora, and the Athymic State on Gastrointestinal Colonization and Infection of BA1B/c mice with Candida albicans," *Infection and Immunity* pp. 764-74, Mar., 1979.

19. Galland, L.; *SuperImmunity for Kids,* E.P. Dutton, New York, p. 215, 1988.

20. Flores, E.C.; Plumb, S.C.; McNeese, M.C.; "Intestinal Parasitosis in an Urban Pediatric Clinic Population," *Am. J. Dis. Child.* Vol. 137, pp. 754-756, 1983.

21. Franco, A.; Ferrari, A.; Pagani, M.; Marconi, R.; et al.; "Inhibition of Candidiacidal Activity of Human Neutrophil Leukocytes by Aminoglycoside Antibiotics," *Antimicrobial Agents and Chemotherapy* pp. 87-88, Jan., 1980.

22. Belsheim, J.A.; Gnarpe, G.H.; "Antibiotics and Granulocytes; Direct and Indirect Effects on Granulocyte Chemotaxis," *Acta. Path. Mocrobiol. Scand.* Sect C, 89:217:221, 1981.

23. *Journal of Antimicrobial Chemotherapy,* 13:413, 1984.

24. Roszkowski, W.; Ko, H.L.; Toszkowski, K.; et al.; "Antibiotics and Immunomodulation: Effects of Cefotaxime, Amikacin, Mezlocillin, Piperacillin, and Clindamycin," *Med. Microbiol. Immunol.* 173:279-289, 1985.

25. Ibid.

26. Berg, R.D.; "Promotion of the Translocation of Enteric Bacteria from the Gastrointestinal Tracts of Mice by Oral Treatment with Penicillin, Clindamycin, or Metronidazole," *Infection and Immunity* pp. 854-861, Sept., 1981.

27. Roe, D.; *Drug-Induced Nutritional Deficiencies,* AVI Publishing, Westport, Connecticut, 1976.

28. Healy, G.B.; "Antimicrobial Therapy of Chronic Otitis Media with Effusion," *Int. J. Ped. Otolar.* 8:13-17, 1984.

29. Mandel, E.M.; Rockette, H.E.; Bluestone, C.D.; Paradise, J.L.; Nozza, R.J.; "Efficacy of Amoxicillin with and without Decongestant-Antihistamine for Otitis Media with Effusion in Children: Results of a Double-blind, Randomized Trial," *New Engl. J. Med.* 316:432-437, 1987.

30. Laxdal, O.E.; Merida, J.; Jones, R.H.T.: "Treatment of Acute Otitis Media: A Controlled Study of 142 Children," *Can. Med. Assoc. J.* 102:263, 1970.

31. Diamant, M.; Diamant, B.; "Abuse and Timing of Use of Antibiotics in Acute Otitis Media," *Arch. Otolaryngol.* 100:226-232, 1974.

32. Shurin, P.A.; Pelton, S.I.; Donner, A.; et al.; "Persistence of Middle Ear Effusion after Acute Otitis Media in Children," *New Engl. J. Med.* 300: 1121, 1979.

33. Thomsen, J.; Meistrup-Larson, K.I.; Sorensen, H.; et al.; "Penicillin and Acute Otitis: Short- and Long-Term Results," *Ann. Otol. Laryngol.* 89 Suppl. 68:271, 1980.

34. Lorentzen, P.; Haugsten, P.; "Treatment of Acute Suppurative Otitis Media," *J. Laryngol.* 91:331, 1977.

35. Froom J.; Culpepper, L.; et al.; "Diagnosis and Antibiotic Treatment of Acute Otitis Media: Report from International Primary Care Network," *Br. Med. J.* 300:582-6, 1990.

36. Schwartz, R.H.; Rodriquez, W.J.; Grundfast, K.; "Pharmacologic Compliance with Antibiotic Therapy for Acute Otitis Media: Influence on Subsequent Middle Ear Effusion," *Pediatrics* Vol. 68 No. 5, Nov., 1981.

37. Meistrup-Larsen, K.I.; Sorensen, H.; et al.; "Two Versus Seven Days Penicillin Treatment for Acute Otitis Media: A Placebo Controlled Trial in Children," *Acta. Otolaryngol.* 96:99-104, 1983.

38. Hendrickse, W.A.; Kusmiesz, H.; et al.; "Five *vs.* Ten Days of Therapy for Acute Otitis Media," *Pediatr. Infect. Dis. J.* 7:14-23, 1988.

39. Chaput de Saintonge, D.M.; Levine, D.F.; "Trial of Three-Day and Ten-Day Courses of Amoxycillin in Otitis Media," *Br. Med. J.* Vol. 284, Apr. 10, 1982.

40. Bain, J.; Murphy, E.; Ross, F.; "Acute Otitis Media: Clinical Course Among Children Who Received a Short Course of High Dose Antibiotic," *Br. Med. J.* Vol. 291, Nov. 2, 1985.

41. Van Buchem, F.L.; "Therapy of Acute Otitis Media: Myringotomy, Antibiotics, or Neither? A Double-Blind Study in Children," *Lancet* 883, Oct. 24, 1981.

42. Persico, M.; et al.; "Recurrent Acute Otitis Media—Prophylactic Penicillin Treatment: A Prospective Study—Part I," *Intl. J. Ped. Otolaryngol.* 10:37-46, 1985.

43. Ibid.

44. Paparella, M.M.; "Complications and Sequelae of Otitis Media: State of the Art" in Lim, D.J. (ed.), *Recent Advances in Otitis Media with Effusion,* Burlington, Ontario, Canada, B.C. Decker, Inc., pp. 316-319, 1984.

45. Pichichero, M.E.; Disney, F.A.; Talpey, W.B.; et al.; "Adverse and Beneficial Effects of Immediate Treatment of Group A Beta-Hemolytic Streptococcal Pharyngitis with Penicillin," *Ped. nfect. Dis. J.* 6:635-643, 1987.

46. Cluff, L.E.; Johnson, J.E.; *Clinical Concepts of Infectious Disease,* 2nd ed., Williams & Wilkins, Baltimore, p. 173, 1978.

47. Van Buchem, F.L.; "Therapy of Acute Otitis Media: Myringotomy, Antibiotics, or Neither? A Double-Blind Study in Children," *Lancet* 883, Oct. 24, 1981.

48. Paparella, M.M.; Goycoolea, M.; et al.; "Silent Otitis Media: Clinical Applications," *Laryngoscope* 96:978-985, Sept., 1986.

49. Pfaltz, C.R.; "Complications of Acute Otitis Media in Children," *Adv. Oto-Rhino-Laryng.* Vol. 40, pp. 70-80, 1988.

50. Castle, M.; Wilfet, C.M.; Cate, T.R.; Osterhout, S.; "Antibiotic Use at Duke University Medical Center," *J.A.M.A.* June 27, 1977.

51. Raye, W.; et al.; "Prescribing of Tetracycline to Children Less than 8 Years Old," *J.A.M.A.* 237:2069-74, 1977.

52. *Wall Street Journal*, Oct. 2, 1989.

53. Froom J.; Culpepper, L.; et al.; "Diagnosis and Antibiotic Treatment of Acute Otitis Media: Report from International Primary Care Network," *Br. Med. J.* 300:582-6, 1990.

54. Lappé, M.; *When Antibiotics Fail: Restoring the Ecology of the Body*, North Atlantic Books, Berkeley, California, 1986.

55. Persico, M.; et al.; "Recurrent Acute Otitis Media—Prophylactic Penicillin Treatment: A Prospective Study—Part I," *Intl. J. Ped. Otolaryngol.* 10:37-46, 1985.

56. Tos, M.; Poulson, G.; Borch, J.; "Etiologic Factors in Secretory Otitis Media," *Arch. Otolaryngol.* 105(10), pp. 582-8, Oct., 1979.

57. Principi, N.; et al.; "Prophylaxis of Recurrent Acute Otitis Media and Middle Ear Effusion: Comparison of Amoxicillin with Sulfamethoxazole and Trimethoprim," *Am. J. Dis. Child.* 143:1414, Dec., 1989.

58. Lappé, M.; *When Antibiotics Fail: Restoring the Ecology of the Body*, North Atlantic Books, Berkeley, California, 1986.

59. Novick, R.P.; "Transmission of Bacterial Pathogens from Animals to Man with Special Reference to Antibiotic Resistance," *Drugs in Livestock Feed*, Vol II, Background papers, Office of Technology Assistance, pp. 3-12, June, 1979.

60. Holmberg, S.D.; Osterholm, M.T.; Senger, K.A.; Cohen, M.L.; "Drug-Resistant Salmonella From Animals Fed Antimicrobials," *New Engl. J. Med.* Vol 311, No. 10, Sept. 6, 1984.

61. "Out of Control: Illegal Sulfa Residues In Meat, Milk," FDA, USDA Statistics cited in *The Safe-Food Gazette*, Center for Science in the Public Interest, 1988.

Chapter 3 Tubes: Effectiveness, Hazards, and Complications

1. Mendelsohn, R.S.; *How to Raise a Healthy Child in Spite of Your Doctor*, Contemporary Books, Inc., Chicago, p. 134, 1984.

2. Paradise, J.L.; "On Tympanostomy Tubes; Rationale, Results, Reservations, and Recommendations," *Pediatrics* Vol. 60, No. 1, July, 1977.

3. Barfold, C.; Rosborg, J.; "Secretory Otitis Media: Long-term Observations After Treatment with Grommets," *Arch. Otolaryngol.* 106:553, 1980.

4. Mawson, S.R.; "Tympanic Effusions in Childen: Long-term Results of Treatment by Myringotomy, Aspiration, and Indwelling Tubes," *J. Laryngol. Otol.* 86:105, 1972.

5. Ibid.

6. Kokko, E.; "Chronic Secretory Otitis Media in Children," *Acta. Otolaryngol.* Suppl., 327, pp. 7-44, 1974.

7. Froom, J.; "Clinical Review: Otitis Media," *J. Fam. Prac.* Vol. 15, No. 4:743-770, 1982.

8. Armstrong, B.W.; Armstrong, R.B.; "Chronic Non-Suppurative Otitis Media: Comparison of Tympanstomy Tubes and Medications Versus Ventilation," *Ann. Otol. Rhinol. Laryngol.* 90:533, 1981.

9. Naunton, R.F.; Panel on experience with middle ear ventilating tubes, "Tympanostomy Tubes: The Conservative Approach," *Ann. Otol. Rhinol. Laryngol.* 90:529, 1981.

10. Stickler, G.B.; "The Attack on the Tympanic Membrane," *Pediatrics* Commentary, p. 291, 1984.

11. Brown, M.J.; Richards, S.H.; Ambegaokar, A.G.; "Grommets and Glue Ear: A Five-Year Follow-up of a Controlled Trial," *J. Roy. Soc. Med.* Vol. 71:353-356, 1978.

12. *Dorland's Pocket Medical Dictionary*, Twenty-Second Edition, W.B. Saunders Company, Philadelphia, 1977.

13. Tos, M.; Poulson, G.; "Secretory Otitis Media: Late Results of Treatment With Grommets," *Arch. Otolaryngol.* 102:672, 1976.

14. Lildholdt, T.; "Ventillation Tubes in Secretory Otitis Media,"

Acta. Otolaryngol. Suppl. 398:1, 1983.

15. Mackinnon, D.M.; *J. Otolaryngol. Otol.* 86:881, 1972.

16. Brown, M.J.; Richards, S.H.; Ambegaokar, A.G.; "Grommets and Glue Ear: A Five-Year Follow-up of a Controlled Trial," *J. Roy. Soc. Med.* 71:353, 1978.

17. Kilby, D.; Richards, S.H.; Hart, G.; "Grommets and Glue Ears: Two-Year Results," *J. Laryngol. Otol.* 86:881-888, 1972.

18. Marshak, G.; Neriah, Z.B.; "Adenoidectomy Versus Tympanostomy in Chronic Secretory Otitis Media," *Ann-Otol-Rhinol-Laryngol* [Suppl] 89 (3 Pt 2 Suppl. 68), pp. 316-8, May-June, 1980.

19. To, S.S.; Pahor, A.L.; Robin, P.E.; "A Prospective Trial of Unilateral Grommets for Bilateral Secretory Otitis Media in Children," *Clin. Otolaryngol.* 9(2):115-117, Apr., 1984.

20. Yanagihara, N.; Yagi, T.; "Limitation of Long-term Ventilation Tube: In View of Complications and Hearing Restoration," *Auris Nasus Larynx* 112 Suppl. 1:s244-6, 1985.

21. Eichenwald, H.; "Otitis Media in the Child," *Hospital Practice* May 30, 1985.

22. Herzon, F.; "Tympanostomy Tubes: Infectious Complications," *Arch. Otolaryngol.* Vol. 106, Oct., 1980.

23. Gates, G.A.; Avery, C.; Prihoda, T.J.; Holt, R.; "Delayed Post-Tympanostomy Otorrhea," *Otolaryngol. Head Neck Surg.* 98:111, 1988.

24. Bluestone, C.D.; Paradise, J.L.; Beery, Q.C.; "Physiology of the Eustachian Tube in the Pathogenesis and Management of Middle Ear Effusions," *Laryngoscope* 82:1654, 1972.

25. Tos, M.; Poulson, G.; "Secretory Otitis Media: Late Results of Treatment With Grommets," *Arch. Otolaryngol.* 102:672, 1976.

26. Grundfast, K.M.; "Complications of Tympanostomy," *Ped. News* Jan., 1981.

27. Tos, M.; Poulson, G.; "Secretory Otitis Media: Late Results of Treatment With Grommets," *Arch. Otolaryngol.* 102:672, 1976.

28. Paradise, J.L.; "Management of Secretory Otitis Media: State of the Art," *Adv. Oto-Rhino-Laryng.* Vol. 40, pp. 99-109, 1988.

Chapter 4 Hearing Loss and Delayed Development: Myth or Reality?

1. Paradise, J.L.; "Otitis Media During Early Life: How Hazardous to Development? A Critical Review of the Evidence," *Pediatrics* Vol. 68, No. 6, Dec., 1981.

2. Bluestone, C.D.; Beery, Q.C.; Paradise, J.L.; "Audiometry and Tympanometry in Relation to Middle-Ear Effusions in Children," *Laryngoscope* 83:594, 1973.

3. Mendelsohn, R.S.; "Ear Infections . . . Tubes in Ears . . . Ear Noises," *The People's Doctor* Vol. 5, No. 5, 1985.

4. Brooks, D.N.; "Otitis Media With Effusion and Academic Attainment" *Intl. J. Ped. Otorhinolaryngol.* 12:39-47, 1986.

5. Roberts, J.E.; Sanyai, M.A.; Burchinal, M.R.; et al.; "Otitis Media in Early Childhood and its Relationship to Later Verbal and Academic Performance," *Pediatrics* Vol. 78, No. 3, Sept., 1986.

6. Kirkwood, C.R.; Kirkwood, M.E.; "Otitis Media and Learning Disabilities: The Case for a Causal Relationship," *J. Fam. Prac.* Vol. 17, No. 2:219-227, 1983.

7. Paradise, J.L.; "Management of Secretory Otitis Media: State of the Art," *Adv. Oto-Rhino-Laryng.* Vol. 40, pp. 99-109, 1988.

8. Paradise, J.L.; "Otitis Media During Early Life: How Hazardous to Development? A Critical Review of the Evidence," *Pediatrics* Vol. 68, No. 6, Dec., 1981.

9. Zinkus, P.W.; Gottlieb, M.I.; Schapiro, M.; "Developmental and Psychoeducational Sequelae of Chronic Otitis Media," *Am. J. Dis. Child.* 132:1100, 1978.

10. Dalzell, J.; Owrid, H.L.; "Children with Conductive Deafness: A Follow-up Study," *Brit. J. Audiol.* 10:87, 1976.

11. Roberts, J.E.; Burchinal, M.R.; et al.; "Otitis Media in Early Childhood and Cognitive, Academic, and Classroom Performance of the School-Aged Child," *Pediatrics* Vol. 83, No. 4, Apr., 1989.

12. Paradise, J.L.; "Otitis Media During Early Life: How Hazardous to Development? A Critical Review of the Evidence," *Pediatrics* Vol. 68, No. 6, Dec., 1981.

Chapter 5 Causes of Childhood Ear Infections

Allergy

1. Morris, W. (ed); *The American Heritage Dictionary of the English Language*, New College Edition, Houghton Mifflin Company, Boston, 1976.

2. *Amino Acids: Metaboism and Medical Applications*, G.L. Blackburn, J.P. Grant and V.R. Young, eds., John Wright-PSG, Inc., Littleton, Massachusetts, 1983.

3. Draper, W.L.; "Secretory Otitis Media," *Clinical Ecology*, Dickey, L. (Ed.), Charles Thomas, Springfield, Illinois, pp. 176-178, 1976.

4. Crook, W.G.; *Are You Allergic: A Guide to Normal Living for Allergic Adults and Children*, Professional Books, Jackson, Tennessee, 1974.

5. Draper, W.L.; "Secretory Otitis Media in Children: A Study of 540 Children," *Laryngoscope* 77:636, 1967.

6. Draper, W.L.; "The Otolaryngologist and the Allergic Child," *South. Med. J.* 59:217, 1966.

7. Bierman, C.W.; Pierson, W.E.; Donaldson, J.A.; "The Evaluation of Middle Ear Function in Children," *Am. J. Dis. Child.* 120:233-6, 1970.

8. Jordan, R.E.; "Role of Allergy in Otology," *Arch. Otolaryngol.* 55:363, 1952.

9. Derlacki, E.L.; Shambaugh, G.E., Jr.; "Allergic Management of Ear Conditions," *Trans. Am. Acad. Ophthalmol. Otolaryngol.* 57:304, 1953.

10. Pang, L.Q.; "The Importance of Allergy in Otolaryngology," *Clinical Ecology,* Dickey, L. (Ed.), Charles Thomas, Springfield, Illinois, pp. 633, 1976.

11. Heiner, D.C., "Respiratory Diseases and Food Allergy," *Ann. Allergy* 53(6 pt 2). pp. 657-64, Dec., 1984 (Review).

12. Rapp, D.; "Management of allergy-related serous otitis," *Am. J. Otol.* 5(6). pp. 463-7, Oct., 1984.

13. Shambaugh, G.E., Jr.; "Serous Otitis: Are Tubes the Answer ?" Paper presented at a meeting of the Society for Clinical Ecology and Environmental Medicine, held concurrently with the annual meeting of the American Academy of Pediatrics (New York, Oct., 24, 1982).

14. O'Connor, R.D.; Ort, H.; Leong, A.B.; Cook, D.A.; Street, D.; Hamburger, R.N.; "Tympanometric Changes Following Nasal Antigen Challenge in Children with Allergic Rhinitis," *Ann. Allergy* 53(6). pp. 468-71, Dec., 1984.

15. Ackerman, M.N.; Friedman, R.A.; Daoyle, W.J.; Bluestone, C.D.; Fireman, P.; "Antigen-Induced Eustachian Tube Obstruction: An Intranasal Provocative Challenge Test," *J. Allergy Clin. Immunol.* 73(5 pt 1), pp. 604-9, May, 1984.

16. McGovern, J.P.; Haywood, T.J.; Fernandez, A.A.; "Allergy and Secretory Otitis Media: An Analysis of 512 Cases," *J.A.M.A.* 200:124-8, 1967.

17. Ruokonen, J.; Paganus, A.; Lehti, H.; "Elimination Diets in the Treatment of Secretory Otitis Media," *Intl. J. Ped. Otorhinolaryngol.* 4:39-46, 1982.

18. Jung, T.T.K.; Giebink, G.S.; Juhn, S.K.; "Effects of Ibuprofen, Corticosteroid, Penicillin on the Pathogenesis of Experimental Pneumococcal Otitis Media," *Recent Advances in Otitis Media with Effusion*, D.J. Lim, C.D. Bluestone, J.O. Klein, et al. (Eds.), B.C. Decker, Inc., Philadelphia, pp. 269-272, 1984.

19. Ojala, K.; Sipila, P.; Sorri, M.; Karma, P.; "Role of Atopic Allergy in Chronic Otitis Media: Valuations Based on Serum IgE and Nasal/Aural Cytologic Findings in Patients with Operated Chronic Ears," *Acta. Otolaryngol.* (Stockh) 93(1-2). pp. 55-60, Jan.-Feb., 1982.

20. Hall, L.J.; Asuncion, J.; Likat, M.; "Allergy Skin Testing Under General Anesthesia with Treatment Response in Ninety-two Patients with Chronic Serous Otitis Media," *Am. J. Otol.* 2(2) pp. 150-7, Oct., 1980.

21. Jaffe, R.; "Evidence for Environmentally Associated Platelet Activation," lecture, American Academy of Medical Preventics, Los Angeles, 1985.

22. Bernstein, J.M.; Ellis, E.; Li, P.; "The Role of IgE-Mediated Hypersensitivity in Otitis Media With Effusion," *Otolaryngol. Head Neck Surg.* 89(5). pp. 874-8, Sept.-Oct., 1981.

23. Pastorello, E.; et al; "Evaluation of Allergic Etiology in Perennial Rhinitis," *Ann. Allergy* 55:854-56, 1985.

24. Folkers, K.; et al.; "Biochemical Evidence for a Deficiency of Vitamin B6 in Subjects Reacting to Monosodium-L-Glutamate by the Chinese Restaurant Syndrome," *Biochem. Biophys. Res. Commun.* 100:972-7, 1981.

25. Papaioannou, R.; Pfeiffer, C.C.; "Sulfite Sensitivity—Unrecognized Threat: Is Molybdenum the Cause?" *J. Orthomol. Psychiat.* 105-110, 1984.

26. Speer, F.; *Food Allergy*, PSG Publishing Co. Inc., Littleton, Mass., (2nd Edition), 1983.

27. Kuvaeva, I.; "The Microecology of the Gastrointestinal Tract and the Immunological Status Under Food Allergy," *Nahrung* 28(6-7):689-93, 1984.

28. Kraemer, M.J.; Richardson, M.A.; Weiss, N.S.; Furukawa, C.T.; Shapiro, G.G.; Rierson, W.E.; Bierman, C.W.; "Risk Factors for Persistent Middle Ear Effusions: Otitis Media, Catarrh, Cigarette Smoke Exposure, and Atopy." *J.A.M.A..* 249(8). pp. 1022-5, Feb. 25, 1983.

29. Bonham G.S.; Wilson, R.W.; "Children's Health in Families with Cigarette Smokers," *Am. J. Publ. Hlth.* 71:290-293, 1981.

30. Ibid, pp. 290-293.

31. Pryor, W.A.; Lightsey, J.W.; Prier, D.G.; "The Production of Free Radicals *in vivo* from the Action of Xenobiotics: The Initiation of Auto-oxidation of Polyunsaturated Fatty Acids by Nitrogen Dioxide and Ozone," *Lipid Peroxides in Biology and Medicine*, New York, Academic Press, pp. 1-22, 1982.

32. National Research Council Committee on Indoor Pollutants, *Indoor Pollutants,* : National Academy Press, Washington, D.C., 1981.

33. Wharton, G.W., "Mites and Commercial Extracts of House Dust" *Science* 6, p. 1382, Mar., 1970.

34. Thatcher, R.W.; "Nutrition, Environmental Toxins and Cognitive Function," lecture, American Academy of Medical Preventics, Los Angeles, 1985.

35. Hartwell, T.D.; Zelon, H.S.; et al.; "Comparative Statistical Analysis for Volatile Halocarbons in Indoor and Outdoor Air," *Indoor Air*, Vol. 4, pp. 57-62, Swedish Council for Building Research, Stockholm, Sweden, 1984.

36. Rosenweig, M.; Hartwell, T.D.; " Statistical Analysis and Evaluation of the Halocarbon Survey," Research Triangle Institute, Final Report, EPA Contract #68-01-5848, 1983.

37. Wallace, L.; Pellizzari, E.; et al.; "Exposure to Volatile Organic Compounds: Direct Measurement in Breathing-Zone Air, Drinking Water, Food, and Exhaled Breath," *Env. Res.* 35:193-211, 1984.

38. Gammage, R.B.; White, D.A.; Gupta, K.C.; "Residential Measurements of High Volatility Organics and Their Sources," *Indoor Air*, Vol. 4, pp. 157-162, Swedish Council for Building Research, Stockholm, Sweden, 1984.

39. Molhave, L.; Moller, J.; "The Atmospheric Environment in Modern Danish Dwellings: Measurements in 39 Flats," *Indoor Climate*, pp. 171-186, Danish Building Research Institute, Copenhagen, 1979.

40. Jarke, F.J.; *ASHRAE Rp 183*, IITRI, Chicago, 1979.

41. Lebret, E.; Van de Wiel, A.; et al.; "Volatile Hydrocarbons in Dutch Homes," *Indoor Air*, Vol 4 pp. 169-174, Swedish Council for Building Research, Stockholm, Sweden, 1984.

42. Seifert, B.; Abraham, H.J.; "Indoor Air Concentrations of Benzene and Some Other Aromatic Hydrocarbons," *Ecotoxicol. Env. Safety* 6: pp. 190-192 1982.

43. Gammage, R.B.; Kaye, S.V.; *Indoor Air and Human Health*, 2nd printing, Lewis Publishers, Chelsea, Michigan, 1985.

44. Ibid.

45. Sterling, D.A.; "Volatile Organic Compounds in Indoor Air: An Overview of Sources, Concentrations, and Health Effects," *Indoor Air and Human Health*, ed. by Gammage, R.B., and Kaye, S.V., Lewis Publishers, Inc., Chelsea, MI, 1984.

46. Molhave, L.; "The Relation Between Emission Rate of Organic Gases, etc, from Building Materials and Their Concentrations in the Indoor Environment," *6th World Congress on Air Quality.* Vol. 2; 345-352, Paris, 1983.

47. Landrigan, P.; *American Academy of Pediatrics*, report to Congress, 1989.

48. Atherton, D.J.; "Breast Feeding and Atopic Eczema," *The British Medical Journal* pp. 775-6, , Sept. 17, 1983.

Infection

49. Froom, J.; "Otitis Media: Clinical Review," *J. Fam. Pract.* Vol. 15, No 4:743-770, 1982.

50. Howie, V.M.; Ploussard, J.H.; Lester, R.L.; "Otitis Media: A Clinical and Bacteriological Correlation," *Pediatrics* 45:29, 1970.

51. Klein, J.O.; "Microbiology of Otitis Media," *Ann. Otol. Rhinol. Laryngol.* 89 (Suppl. 68):98, 1980.

52. Asman, B.J.; Fireman, P.; "The Role of Allergies in the Development of Otitis Media with Effusion," *Intl. Ped.* Vol. 3, No 3, July-Sept., 1988.

53. Adlington, P.; Hooper, W.K.; "Virus Studies in Secretory Otitis Media," *J. Laryngol. Otol.* 94:191, 1980.

54. Klein, J.O.; "Microbiology of Otitis Media," *Ann. Otol. Rhinol. Laryngol.* 89 (Suppl. 68):98, 1980.

55. Asman, B.J.; Fireman, P.; "The Role of Allergies in the Development of Otitis Media with Effusion," *Intl. Ped.* Vol. 3, No. 3, July-Sept., 1988.

56. Pelton, S.I.; Teele, D.W.; Shurin, P.A.; et al.; "Disparate Cultures of Middle Ear Fluids," *Am. J. Dis. Child.* 134:951, 1980.

57. Schwartz, R.; Rodriguez, W.; et al.; "The Increasing Incidence of Ampicillin-Resistant *Haemophilus influenzae:* A Cause of Otitis Media," *J.A.M.A.* Vol. 239, No. 4, Jan. 23, 1978.

58. Chandra, R.K.; "Trace Element Regulation of Immunity and Infection," *Am. J. Clin. Nutr.* 35:417-68 (Suppl.), 1985.

59. Bondestam, M.; Foucard, T.; Gebre-Medhin, M.; "Subclinical Trace Element Deficiency in Children with Undue Susceptibility to Infections," *Act. Paed. Sc.* 74:515-520, 1985.

60. Golden, M.; Jackson, A.; Golden, B.; "Effect of Zinc on Thymus of Recently Malnourished Children," *Lancet*, ii, pp. 1057-9, 1977.

61. Beisel, W.R.; "Single Nutrients and Immunity," *Am. J. Clin. Nutr.* 35:417-68 (Suppl.), 1982.

62. Werbach, M.R.; *Nutritional Influences on Illness: A Sourcebook of Clinical Research*, Third Line Press, Inc., Tarzana, CA, p. 252, 1987.

63. Beach, R.; Gershwin, M.; Hurley, L.; "Persistent Immunological Consequences of Gestational Zinc Deprivation," *Am. J. Clin. Nutr.* 38:579-90, 1983.

64. Sanchez, A.; et al.; "Role of Sugars in Human Neutrophilic Phagocytosis," *Am. J. Clin. Nutr.* 26:180, 1973.

65. Teele, D.W.; Pelton, S.I.; Klein, J.O.; "Bacteriology of Acute Otitis Media Unresponsive to Initial Antimicrobial Therapy," *J. Pediatr.* 98:537, 1981.

66. Skoner, D.P.; Stillwagon, P.K.; et al.; "Inflammatory Mediators in Chronic Otitis Media with Effusion," *Arch. Otolaryngol. Head Neck Surg.* Vol. 114, pp. 1131-1133, Oct., 1988.

67. Jung, T.T.K.; "Prostaglandins, Leukotrienes, and Other Arachidonic Acid Metabolites in the Pathogenesis of Otitis Media," *Laryngoscope* 98, Sept., 1988.

Mechanical Obstruction

68. Ford, F.R.; "Breech Delivery in its Possible Relations to Injury of the Spinal Cord with Special Reference to Infantile Paraplegia," *Arch. Neurol. Psychiat.* 14, 742, 1925.

69. Towbin, A.; "Latent Spinal Cord and Brain Stem Injury in Newborn Infants," *Develop. Med. Child. Neurol.* 11, pp. 54-68, 1969.

70. Duncan, J.M.; "Laboratory Note: On the Tensile Strength of the Fresh Adult Foetus," *Brit. Med. J.* ii, 763, 1874.

71. Frymann, V.; "Relations of Disturbances of Cranio-sacral Mechanisms to Symptomatology of the Newborn," *J. Am. Osteopathic Assoc.* 65:1059, 1966.

72. Gutmann, G.; "Das Atlas-Blockierungs-Syndrome des Sauglings und des Kleinkindes," *Manuelle Med.* 25:5-10, 1987.

73. Peters, R.E.; Chance, M.E.; "A Priceless Legacy-Lost, Strayed or Forfeited?" *J. Austral. Chiropr. Assoc.* Vol. 18, No. 3, pp. 81-84, Sept., 1988.

74. Chapman-Smith, D.; "Blocked Atlantal Nerve Syndrome in Babies and Infants," *The Chiropractic Report* Vol. 3, No. 2., Jan., 1989 (a review of Peters & Chance, and Gutmann is provided).

75. Brennan, P.C.; Hondras, M.A.; "Priming of Neutrophils for Enhanced Respiratory Burst by Manipulation of the Thoracic Spine," *Proceedings of the International Conference on Spinal Manipulation* pp. 160-163, Mar. 31-Apr. 1,1989.

76. Gutmann, G; "Das Atlas-Blockierungs-Syndrome des Sauglings und des Kleinkindes," *Manuelle Med.* 25:5-10, 1987.

77. Winsor, H.; "Sympathetic Segmental Disturbances - II; The Evidences of the Association, in Dissected Cadavers, of Visceral Disease With Vertebral Deformities of the Same Segments," *Med. Times* 49:1-7, 1921.

78. Suh, C.H.; Professor and Chairman, Department of Engineering Design and Evaluation, University of Colorado, Boulder, Colorado.

79. Seifert, J.; "Die Kopfgelenksblockierung des Neugeborenen," In: Lewit, K., Gutmann, G. (eds), *Rehabilitacia*, Prague: Bratislawa, Vol. 8, 53, 1975.

Nutrition

80. Rudin, D.O.; "Omega-3 Essential Fatty Acids in Medicine," *1984-1985 Yearbook of Nutritional Medicine*, Bland, J.S. (Ed.), Keats Publishing, New Canaan, Connecticut, p. 41, 1985.

81. Ibid, p. 42.

82. Rudin, D.O.; Felix, C.; *The Omega-3 Phenomenon*, Avon Books, New York, 1987.

83. Ibid, p. 22.

84. Moser, P.; Reynolds, R.; "Dietary Zinc Intake and Zinc Concentrations of Plasma, Erythrocytes, and Breastmilk in Antepartum and Postpartum Lactating and Non-Lactating Women: A Longitudinal Study," *Am. J. Clin. Nut.* 38:101-108, 1983.

85. Holman, R.T.; Johnson, S.; Hatch, T.F.; "A Case of Human Linolenic Acid Deficiency Involving Neurological Abnormalities," *Am. J. Clin. Nutr.* 35:617-23, 1982.

86. Enig, M.G.; Pallansch, L.A.; Sampugna, J.; Keeney, M.; "Fatty Acid Composition of the Fat in Selected Food Items With Emphasis on Trans Components," *J. Am. Oil Chem. Soc.* 60:1788-1795, 1983.

87. "Trans Fatty Acids in Foods," *Nutrition Reviews* Vol. 42, No. 8, 1984.

88. Erasmus, U.; *Fats and Oils: The Complete Guide to Fats and Oils in Health and Nutrition*, Alive Books, Vancouver, Canada, 1986.

89. "Trans Fatty Acids in Foods," *Nutrition Reviews* Vol. 42, No. 8, 1984.

90. Enig, M.G.; Pallansch, L.A.; Sampugna, J.; Keeney, M.; "Fatty Acid Composition of the Fat in Selected Food Items With Emphasis on Trans Components," *J. Am. Oil Chem. Soc.* 60:1788-1795, 1983.

91. Horrobin, D.F.; "Essential Fatty Acids: a review," in *Clinical Uses of Essential Fatty Acids* , Eden Press, New York, pp. 3-31, 1982.

92. Berkson, D.; "Nutritional Considerations for Female Health Problems," lecture on clinical nutrition presented in Bloomington, Minnesota, Nov., 1987.

93. Ibid.

94. Rudin, D.O.; "Omega-3 Essential Fatty Acids in Medicine," *1984-1985 Yearbook of Nutritional Medicine*, Bland, JS (Ed.), Keats Publishing, New Canaan, Connecticut, p. 41, 1985.

95. Pennington, J.A.T.; Young, B.E.; et al.; "Mineral Content of Foods and Total Diets: The Selected Minerals in Foods Survey, 1982 to 1984," Food and Drug Administration, Kansas City, Missouri.

96. Chole, R.A.; "Squamous Metaplasia of the Middle Ear Mucosa During Vitamin A Deprivation," *Otolaryngol. Head Neck Surg.* 87(6):837-44, Nov.-Dec., 1979.

97. Golden, M.; Jackson, A.; Golden, B.; "Effect of Zinc on Thymus of Recently Malnourished Children," *Lancet* ii, pp. 1057-9, 1977.

98. Bondestam, M.; Foucard, T.; Gebre-Medhin, M.; "Subclnical Trace Element Deficiency in Children with Undue Susceptibility to Infections," *Act. Paed. Sc.* 74:515-520, 1985.

99. Manku, M.S.; et al.; "Reduced Levels of Prostaglandin Precursors in the Blood of Atopic Patients: Defective Delta-6-Desaturase Function as a Biochemical Basis for Atopy," *Prostaglandins, Leukotrienes in Medicine* 9:615-28, 1982.

100. Galland, L.; "Increased Requirements for Essential Fatty Acids in Atopic Individuals: A Review with Clinical Descriptions," *J. Am. Col. Nutr.* 5:213-28, 1986.

101. Skoner, D.P.; Stillwagon, P.K.; et al.; "Inflammatory Mediators in Chronic Otitis Media with Effusion," *Arch. Otolaryngol. Head Neck Surg.* Vol. 114, pp. 1131-1133, Oct., 1988.

102. Jung, T.T.K.; "Prostaglandins, Leukotrienes, and Other Arachidonic Acid Metabolites in the Pathogenesis of Otitis Media," *Laryngoscope* 98: Sept., 1988.

103. Stenmark, K.R.; James, S.L.; et al.; "Leukotriene C4 and D4 in Neonates with Hypoxemia and Pulmonary Hypertension," *New Engl. J. Med.* 309:77, 1983.

104. Goldman, D.W.; Goetzl, E.J.; "Mediation and Modulation of Immediate Hypersensitivity and Inflammation by Products of the Oxygenation of Arachidonic Acid," *Immunology of Inflammation*, P.A. Ward, (Ed.) Elsevier Science Pub., New York, pp. 163-187, 1976.

105. Dahlen, S.; Sammuelsson, B.; "Leukotrienes are Potent Constrictors of Human Bronchi," *Nature* 288:484, 1980.

106. Hanna, C.J.; Bach, M.K.; et al.; "Slow-reacting Leukotrienes and Pulmonary Vascular Smooth Muscle in vitro," *Nature* 210:343,1981.

107. Jung, T.T.K.; "Prostaglandins, Leukotrienes, and Other Arachidonic Acid Metabolites in the Pathogenesis of Otitis Media," *Laryngoscope* 98: Sept., 1988.

108. Smith, D.M.; Jung, T.T.K.; Juhn, S.K.; Berlinger, N.T.; Gerrard, J.M.; "Prostaglandins in Experimental Otitis Media," *Arch. Otorhinolaryngol.* 225:207-9, 1979.

109. Skoner, D.P.; Stillwagon, P.K.; et al.; "Inflammatory Mediators in Chronic Otitis Media with Effusion," *Arch. Otolaryngol. Head Neck Surg.* Vol. 114, pp. 1131-1133, Oct., 1988.

110. Jung, T.T.K.; Giebink, G.S.; Juhn, S.K.; "Effects of Ibuprofen, Corticosteroid, Penicillin on the Pathogenesis of Experimental Pneumococcal Otitis Media," *Recent Advances in Otitis Media with Effusion* , D.J. Lim, C.D. Bluestone, J.O. Klein, et al. (Eds.), B.C. Decker, Inc., Philadelphia, pp. 269-272, 1984.

111. Roe, D.; *Drug-Induced Nutritional Deficiency,* AVI Publishing Co., Westport, Connecticut, 1976.

Chapter 6 Home Care for Earaches

1. Wootan, G.; "Home-Care for Children," *Mothering* Winter, p. 38, 1985.

2. Moskowitz, R.; "Unvaccinated Children," *Mothering* Winter, 1987.

3. Cummings, S.; Ullman, D.; *Everybody's Guide to Homeopathic Medicines*, Jeremy P. Tarcher, Los Angeles, p. 113, 1984.

4. Thompson, L.L.; "Fear of Fever is Often Worse Than Fever Itself," *Washington Post* Review reprinted in the *Minneapolis Star Tribune* Nov. 10, 1989.

5. Nelson, K.B.; Ellenberg, J.H.; "Prognosis in Children with Febrile Seizures," *Pediatrics* May, 1978; Schmitt, B. D.; "Fever Phobia," *Am. J. Dis. of Child.* pp. 176-186, Feb., 1980.

6. Mendelsohn, R.S.; *How to Raise a Healthy Child in Spite of Your Doctor*, Contemporary Books, Inc., Chicago, pp. 66-79, 1984.

7. Carmichael, L.E.; Barnes, F.D.; Percy, D.H.; "Temperature as a Factor in Resistance of Young Puppies," *J. Infect. Dis.* 120:669, 1969.

8. Kluger, M.J.; "Fever," *Pediatrics* 66:720-724, 1980.

9. Kluger, M.J.; Rothenberg, B.A.; "Fever and Reduced Iron: Their Interaction as a Host Defense Response to Bacterial Infection," *Science* 203:374, 1979.

10. Schmitt, B.D.; "Fever Phobia," *Am. J. Dis. Child.* pp. 176-186, Feb., 1980.

11. Nelson, K.B.; Ellenberg, J.H.; "Prognosis in Children with Febrile Seizures," *Pediatrics* May, 1978.

12. Mendelsohn, R.S.; *How to Raise a Healthy Child in Spite of Your Doctor*, Contemporary Books, Inc., Chicago, pp. 75, 1984.

13. Doran, T.F.; DeAngelis, C.; Baumgardner, R.A.; Mellitis, E.D.; "Acetaminophen: More Harm Than Good for Chickenpox?" *J. Pediatrics* 114(6):1045-8, 1989.

14. Mendelsohn, R.S.; *How to Raise a Healthy Child in Spite of Your Doctor*, Contemporary Books, Inc., Chicago, p. 69, 1984.

15. Ibid, pp. 78-79.

16. Meduski, J.W.; *Practical Guidelines for the Selection and Application of Lactobacilli and Bifidobacteria in Preventive Medicine and Therapy*, unpublished guidelines, 1988.

17. Bjorkstein, B.; Back, O.; Gustavson, K.; et al.; "Zinc and Immune Function in Down's Syndrome," *Acta. Paediatr. Scand.* 69:183-187, 1980.

18. "Correction of Impaired Immunity in Down's Syndrome by Zinc," *Nutrition Reviews* 38;11:365-7, 1980.

19. Rowe, A.H.; *Clinical Allergy*, Philadelphia, Lea and Febiger, 1937.

20. Crook W.G.; *The Yeast Connection,* Professional Books, Jackson, Tennessee, pp. 18-26, 1985.

21. Ibid, p. 77.

22. Florey, H.W.; *British Medical Journal* p. 654, 1943.

23. Chedid, L.; Parent, M.; Boyer, F.; Skarnes, R.C.; "Non-Specific Host Response in Tolerance to the Lethal Effect of Endotoxin," *Bacterial Endotoxins,* M. Landy and W. Braun, (eds.), Rutgers, the State University, p. 112, 1964.

24. Boswinkel, J.C.; The effects of homeopathic dilutions of DDVP on locusts in the Northwestern Sahara, Personal communication, 1989.

25. Riley, D.T.; Taylor, M.A.; "Is Homeopathy a Placebo Response: Controlled Trial of Homeopathic Potency, with Pollen in Hayfever as Model," *Lancet* pp. 881-886, Oct. 18, 1986.

26. Moessinger, P.; "Zur Behandlung der Otitis Media mit Pulsatilla," *Allgemeine Homoopathische Zeitung* 230:89, 1985.

27. Neustaedter, R.; "Management of Otitis Media with Effusion in Homeopathic Practice," *J. Am. Inst. Homeop.* Vol. 79, Nos. 3 and 4, 1986.

28. Cummings, S.; Ullman, D.; *Everybody's Guide to Homeopathic Medicines*, Jeremy P. Tarcher, Los Angeles, pp. 41-42, 1984.

29. Chapman-Smith, D.; "Blocked Atlantal Nerve Syndrome in Babies and Infants," *The Chiropractic Report*, Jan., 1989, Vol. 3, No. 2 (a review of Peters & Chance, and Gutmann is provided).

30. Gutmann, G.; "Das Atlas-Blockierungs-Syndrome des Sauglings und des Kleinkindes," *Manuelle Med.* 25:5-10, 1987.

31. Hoffman, D.; *The Holistic Herbal*, The Findhorn Press, Findhorn, Moray, Scotland, 1983.

32. Meruelo, D.; et al.; *Proceedings of the National Academy of Sciences*, Vol. 85, pp. 5230-4, July, 1988.

33. *The Biology and Cultivation of Edible Mushrooms*, Chang and Hayes, (eds.), Academic Press, Inc., pp. 169-187, 1978.

34. Salmi, H.A.; Sarne, S.; *Effects of Silymarin on Chemical, Functional, and Morphological Alterations of the Liver: A Double-Blind, Placebo-Controlled Study*, Central Military Hospital-1, Dept. of Public Health, Helsinki, Finland, Sept. 25, 1981.

35. Ikeda, K.; Takasaka, T.; "Treatment of Secretory Otitis Media with Kampo Medicine," *Arch. Otorhinolaryngol.* 245:234-236, 1988.

36. Benedict, M.; Personal communication, 1989.

37. "Echinacea," *Medical Nutrition* Vol. 4, No. 2, pp.14-16, 1989.

38. Rasic, J.L.; Kurman, J.A.; *Bifidobacteria and Their Role*, Birkhauser Verlag, Basel-Boston-Stuttgart, 1983.

39. Speck, P.; Gilliland, A.; "Antagonisitc Action of L. Acidophilus Toward Intestinal and Foodborne Pathogens in Associative Cultures," *J. Food Prot.* Vol. 40, No. 12, pp. 820-823, 1977.

40. Shahani, K.M.; Hathaway, I.L.; and Kelly, P.L.; "B-complex Vitamin Content of Cheese. II Niacin, Pantothenic Acid, Pyridoxine, Biotin & Folic Acid," *J. Dairy Sci.* 45:833, 1962.

41. Shahani, K.M.; Kilara, A.; "Lactase Activity of Cultured and Acidified Dairy Products," *J. Dairy Sci.* 59:2031, 1976.

42. Dubos, R.; *The Microbiota In Man Adapting,* Yale University Press, New Haven, Connecticut, p. 110, 1965.

43. Goldin, B.; Gorbach, S.L.; "Alterations in Fecal Microflora Enzymes Related to Age, Lactobacili Supplements and Dimethyl Hydrazine," *Cancer* 40:2421, 1977.

44. Ibid.

45. Friend, B.A.; Rarmer, R.E.; Shahani, K.M.; "Effect of Feeding and Intraperitoneal Implantation of Yogurt Culture Cells on Ehrlich Ascites Tumor," *Milchwissenschaff* 37 (12), 1982.

46. Purohit, B.C.; Joshi, K.P.; et al.; "The Formation of Germtubes by Candida albicans, when Grown with Staphylococcus pyogenes, E. coli, Klebsiella pneumoniae, L. acidophilus and Proteus vulgaris," *Mycopathologia* Vol. 62, 3:187-189, 1977.

47. Mayer, J.B.; "Viren Und Darmflora," *Paediat.* Paedol 1:131-137, 1965.

48. Meduski, J.W.; *Practical Guidelines for the Selection and Application of Lactobacilli and Bifidobacteria in Preventive Medicine and Therapy,* unpublished guidelines, 1988.

Chapter 7 Preventing Ear Infections in Your Child

1. Chandra, R.K.; "Prospective Studies of the Effect of Breastfeeding on Incidence of Infection and Allergy," *Acta. Pediatr. Scand.* 68(5), pp. 691-4, Sept., 1979.

2. Ibid.

3. Ibid.

4. Saarinen, U.; "Breastfeeding Prevents Otitis Media," *Nutrition Reviews* Vol. 41, No. 8, p. 241, Aug., 1983.

5. Persico, M.; et al.; "Recurrent Middle-Ear Infections in Infants; The Protective Role of Maternal Breast Feeding," *Ear, Nose, & Throat J.* Vol. 62, June, 1983.

6. Gammage, R.B.; Kaye, S.V.; *Indoor Air and Human Health,* 2nd printing, Lewis Publishers, Chelsea, Michigan, 1985.

7. Kenny, E.; New York Research Laboratory, memo, 1985.

8. Minnesota Department of Health, Memo, 1989.

9. Wald, E.R.; Dashefsky, B.; et al.; "Frequency and Severity of Infections in Day Care," *J. Pediatr.* 112:540-6, 1988.

10. Pickering, L.K.; Woodward, W.E.; "Diarrhea in Day Care Centers," *Ped. Infect. Dis. J.* Vol. 1, No. 1, pp. 47-51, 1982.

11. Schuman, S.; "Day Care Associated Infection: More Than Meets the Eye," *J.A.M.A.* Jan. 7, 1983.

12. Redmond, S.; Pichichero, M.; "*Haemophilus influenzae* Type b Disease: An Epidemiologic Study with Special Reference to Day Care Centers," *J.A.M.A.* Vol. 252, No. 18, pp. 2581-2584, 1984.

13. Black, R.E.; Dykes, A.C.; Sinclair, S.P.; Wells, J.G.; "Giardiasis in Day-Care Centers: Evidence of Person-to-Person Transmission," *Pediatrics* Vol. 60, No. 4, Oct., 1977.

14. Jasper, W.F.; "My Mother the State: But is it Good for Kids?" *The New American* Vol. 5, No. 3, Jan. 30, 1989.

15. Johnson, A.S.; Leibowitz, A.; Waite, L.J.; "Child Care and Children's Illness," *Am. J. Pub. Hlth.* Vol. 78, No. 9, pp. 1175-1177, 1988.

16. Wald, E.R.; Dashefsky, B.; et al.; "Frequency and Severity of Infections in Day Care," *J. Pediatr.* 112:540-6, 1988.

17. Strangert, K.; "Otitis media in Young Children in Different Types of Day Care," *Scand. J. Infect. Dis.* 9:119-23, 1977.

18. Pukander, J.; Sipila, M.; Karma, P.; "Occurrence of and Risk Factors in Acute Otitis Media. In: Lim D.J., Bluestone, D.C., Klein,

J.O., Nelson, J.D., eds. *Recent Advances in Otitis Media With Effusion*, B. C. Decker, Philadelphia, pp. 9-13, 1984.

19. Birch, L.; Elbrond, O.; "Prospective Epidemiological Study of Secretory Otitis Media in Chilren not Attending Kindergarten, An Incidence Study," *Intl. J. Ped. Otorhinolaryngol.* 11, pp. 183-190, 1986.

20. Wald, E. R.; Dashefsky, B.; et al.; "Frequency and Severity of Infections in Day Care," *J. Pediatr.* 112:540-6, 1988.

21. Benedict, M.; Personal Communication, 1989.

22. Cheraskin, E.; "Sucrose, Neutrophilic Phagocytosis and Resistance to Disease," *Dental Survey* 52(12):46-48, 1976.

23. Durlack, J.; *Le Diabete* 19:99-113, 1971.

24. Lindeman, R.D.; et al.; *Magnesium in Health and Disease*, SP Medical and Scientific Books, Jamaica, N. Y., pp. 236-45, 1980.

25. Freundlich, M.; et al.; "Infant Formula as a Cause of Aluminum Toxicity in Neonatal Uremia," *Lancet* 2:527-29, 1985.

26. Pesce; McKean; "Toxic Susceptibilities in the Newborn with Special Consideration with Polysorbate Toxicity," *Ann. Clin. Lab. Sci.* 19:70-73, 1989.

27. "Plasma Aluminum Measurements in Term Infants Fed Human Milk or a Soy-Based Infant Formula," *Pediatrics* Vol. 84, No. 6, pp. 1105-7, Dec., 1989.

28. Galland, L.; Buchman, D.D.; *SuperImmunity for Kids*, E.P. Dutton, New York, 1988.

29. Flaws, B.; "Stagnant Food and Pediatric Disease: The Care and Feeding of Infants According to Traditional Chinese Medicine," *Am. J. Acupunct.* Vol. 17, No. 4, pp. 331-336, 1989.

30. Kozlovsky, A.S.; et al.; "Effects of Diets High in Simple Sugars on Urinary Chromium Losses," *Metabolism* 35:515-18, 1986.

31. Settle, D.M.; Patterson, C.C.; "Lead in Albacore: Guide to Lead Pollution in the Americans," *Science* 207:1167, 1980.

32. Flaws, B.; "Stagnant Food and Pediatric Disease: The Care and Feeding of Infants According to Traditional Chinese Medicine," *Am. J. Acupunct.* Vol. 17, No. 4, pp. 331-336, 1989.

Chapter 8 Alternative Treatment: Some Solutions

1. Akerle, O.; "The Best of Both Worlds: Bringing Traditional Medicine up to Date," *Soc. Sci. Med.* Vol. 24, No. 2, pp. 177-181, 1987.

2. Eisenberg, L.; "Preventive Pediatrics: The Promise and the Peril," *Pediatrics* Vol. 80, No. 3, pp. 415-416, 1987.

3. Ikeda, K.; Takasaka, T.; "Treatment of Secretory Otitis Media with Kampo Medicine," *Arch. Oto-Rhino-Laryngol.* 245:234-236, 1988.

4. Lildholdt, T.; "Unilateral Grommet Insertion and Adenoidectomy in Bilateral Secretory Otitis Media: Preliminary Report of the Results in 91 Children," *Clin. Otolaryngol.* 4:87-93, 1982. The quote appears in a footnote to this paper.

5. Paparella, M.M.; "Complications and Sequelae of Otitis Media: State of the Art," in Lim, D.J. (ed.) *Recent Advances in Otitis Media with Effusion*, B.C. Decker, Inc., Burlingtion, Ontario, Canada, pp. 316-319, 1984.

6. Levine, S.A.; Kidd, P.M.; *Antioxidant Biochemical Adaptation: Doorways to the New Science and Medicine*, Biocurrents Research Corporation, San Fransisco, 1984.

7. Bland, J.S.; Baker, S.M.; *Immune Modulation: The Prevention of Immunosenscence*, HealthComm, Inc., Gig Harbor, WA, 1989.

8. Messer, S.; *Homeopathy & Otitis in Children*, Audio Taped Lecture, Homeopathic Educational Services, Berkeley, California, 1986.

9. Ibid.

10. Ibid.

11. Borland, D.M.; *Children's Types*, World Homeopathic Links, New Dehli-110055.

12. Santwani, M.T.; *Common Ailments of Children and Their Homeopathic Management*, Jain Publishing Co., New Delhi, 1983.

13. Neustaedter, R.; "Management of Otitis Media with Effusion in Homeopathic Practice," *J. Am. Inst. Homeop.* Vol. 79, Nos. 3 & 4, p. 19, 1986.

14. Houghton, H.C.; *Lectures on Clinical Otology*, Otis Clapp & Son, New York Homeopathic Medical College, 1885.

15. Gutmann, G.; and Medizin, M.; "Blocked Atlantal Nerve Syndrome in Babies and Infants," *Manuel Med.* 25; 5-10, 1987.

16. La Francis, M.E.; "A Chiropractic Perspective on Atlantoaxial Instability in Down's Syndrome," *J. Manip. Phys. Therap.* March/April, 1990. (See also, Davidson, R. G.; "Atlantoaxial Instability in Individuals with Down Syndrome: A Fresh Look at the Evidence," *Pediatrics* Vol. 81, No. 6, 1988.)

17. Scott, J.; *The Treatment of Children by Acupuncture*, The Journal of Chinese Medicine, England, 1986.

18. *Essentials of Chinese Acupuncture*, Foreign Languages Press, Beijing, 1980.

19. Becker, R.O.; *Cross Currents: The Perils of Electropollution, The Promise of Electromedicine*, Jeremy P. Tarcher, Inc., Los Angeles, pp. 130-132, 1990.

20. White, A.; Personal communication, 1990.

21. Benedict, M.; Personal communication, 1989.

22. Jung, T.T.K.; "Prostaglandins, Leukotrienes, and Other Arachidonic Acid Metabolites in the Pathogenesis of Otitis Media," *Laryngoscope*, 98: p. 983, Sept., 1988.

23. Proceedings of the National Academy of Sciences, Vol. 86, No. 16, Aug., 1989. Includes a discussion of Ascorbic acid as a free-radical scavenger.

24. Loh, H.S.; Walters, K.; Wilson, C.W.M.; "The Effects of Aspirin on the Metabolic Availability of Ascorbic Acid in Detoxification of Human Beings," *J. Clin. Pharmacol.* 13, p. 480, 1973.

25. Nandi, B.K.; Subramanian, N.; Majumder, A.K.; Chatterjee, I.B.; "Effect of Ascorbic Acid on Detoxification of Histamine Under Stress Conditions," *Biochem. Pharm.* 23, pp. 643-647, 1974.

26. Hausteen, B.; "Flavonoids, a Class of Natural Products of High Pharmacologic Potency," *Biochem. Pharm.* 32:7, pp. 1141-1148, 1983.

27. Voorhees, J.J.; "Leukotrienes and Other Lipoxygenase Products in the Pathogenesis and Therapy of Psoriasis and Other Dermatoses," *Arch. Dermatol.* 119, pp. 541-547, 1983.

28. Srimal, R.C.; Dhawan, B.N.; "Pharmacology of Diferuloyl Methane (Curcumin), a Non-Steroidal Anti-Inflammatory Agent," *J. Pharm. Pharmac.* 25:447-452.

29. Chandra, D.; Gupta, S.S.; "Anti-Inflammatory and Anti-Arthritic Activity of Volatile Oil of *Curcuma longa*," *Indian J. Med. Res.* 60:138-142, 1972.

30. Sharma, S.C.; Mukhtar, H.; et al.; "Lipid Peroxide Formation in Experimental Inflammation," *Biochem. Pharm.* 21:1210-1214, 1972.

31. Salimath, B.P.; Sundaresh, C.S.; Srinivas, L.; "Dietary Components Inhibit Lipid Peroxidation in Erythrocyte Membrane," *Nutr. Res.* 6:1171-1178, 1986.

32. Bauman, J.; Wurn, G.; et al.; "Effect of Quercitin on Prostaglandin Synthetase," *Prostaglandins* 20:627, 1980.

33. Underhill, J.; "Bioflavonoids—Chemistry and Physiology," *Can. J. Biochem. Physiol.* 35:219, 1957.

34. Regtop, H.; "Nutrition, Leukotrienes and Inflammatory Disorders," *1984-85 Yearbook of Nutritional Medicine*, J. Bland (ed.), Keats Publishing, Inc., New Canaan, Connecticut, pp. 55-69, 1985.

35. Flynn, D.L.; et al.; "Inhibition of Human Neutrophil 5-Lipoxygenase Activity by Gingerdione, Shogaoi, Capsaicin and Related Pungent Compounds," *Prost. Leuk. Med.* 24:195-198, 1986.

36. Ikeda, K.; Takasaka, T.; "Treatment of Secretory Otitis Media with Kampo Medicine," *Arch. Oto-Rhino-Laryngol.* 245:234-236, 1988.

37. Gilbert, V.A.; Zebrowski, E.J.; Chan, A.C.; "Differential Effects of Megavitamin E on Prostaglandin and Thromboxane Synthesis in Streptozotocin-Induced Diabetic Rats," *Horm. Metabol. Res.* 15, pp. 320-325, 1983.

38. Voorhees, J.J.; "Leukotrienes and Other Lipoxygenase Products in the Pathogenesis and Therapy of Psoriasis and Other Dermatoses," *Arch. Dermatol.* 119, pp. 541-547, 1983.

39. Chandra, R.K.; "Single Nutrient Deficiency and Cell-Mediated Immunity: Zinc," *Amer. J. Clin. Nutr.* 33:736, 1980.

40. Horrobin, D.; "Gamma-Linolenic Acid in Medicine," *1984-85 Yearbook of Nutritional Medicine*, J. Bland (ed.), Keats Publishing, Inc., New Canaan, Connecticut, p. 30, 1985.

41. Velardo, B.; et al.; "Decrease of Platelet Activity after Intake of Small Amounts of Eicosapentaenoic Acid in Diabetics, " *Throm. Haemostas.* 48:3, p. 344, 1982.

42. Horrobin, D.; "Gamma-Linolenic Acid in Medicine," *1984-85 Yearbook of Nutritional Medicine*, J. Bland (ed.), Keats Publishing, Inc., New Canaan, Connecticut, p. 25, 1985.

43. Smith, D.W.; *Recognizable Patterns of Human Malformation*, 3rd edition, Saunders, Philadelphia, 1982.

44. Clarren, S.K.; Smith, D.W.; "The Fetal Alcohol Syndrome," *New Engl. J. Med.* 198:1063-1067, 1978.

45. Church, M.W.; Gerkin, K.P.; "Hearing Disorders in Children with Fetal Alcohol Syndrome: Findings From Case Reports," *Pediatrics* Vol. 82, No. 2, 1988.

46. Ibid.

47. Chandra, R.K.; "Single Nutrient Deficiency and Cell-Mediated Immunity: Zinc," *Amer. J. Clin. Nutr.* 33:736, 1980.

48. Beisel, W.R.; "Single Nutrients and Immunity," *Am. J. Clin. Nutr.* 35, pp. 449-451 Suppl., Feb., 1982.

49. Allen, J.; Kay, N.; McClain, C.; "Severe Zinc Deficiency in Humans: Association with T-Lymphocyte Dysfunction," *Ann. Int. Med.* 95:154-7, 1981.

50. Golden, M.; Jackson, A.; Golden, B.; "Effect of Zinc on Thymus of Recently Malnourished Children," *Lancet* ii, pp. 1057-9, 1977.

51. Hamblin, J.; Hussain, J.; Akbar, A.; et al.; "Immunological Reason for Chronic Ill Health after Infectious Mononucleosis," *Brit. Med. J.* 287:85-88, 1983.

52. Willmott, F.; Say, J.; Downey, D.; et al.; "Zinc and Recalcitrant Trichomoniasis," *Lancet* i, p. 1053, 1983.

53. Klevay, L.M.; Keck, S.; Bacome, D.F.; "Evidence of Dietary Copper and Zinc Deficiencies," *J.A.M.A.* 241, No. 18, pp. 1916-1918, 1979.

54. Chandra, R.K.; "Trace Element Regulation of Immunity and Infection," *J. Am. Coll. Nutr.* 4(1):5-16, 1985.

55. Kiremidjian-Schumacher, L.; Stotzky, G.; "Selenium and Immune Responses," *Environ. Res.* 42:277-303, 1987.

56. Kidd, P.; "Germanium-132: Homeostatic Normalizer and Immunostimulant—A Review of its Preventive and Therapeutic Efficacy," *Intl. Clin. Nutr. Rev.* Special Article, Vol. 7, No. 1, Jan., 1987.

57. Chandra, R.K.; "Nutrition and Immunity—Basic Considerations," Part 1, *Contemp. Nutr.* 11(11), 1986.

58. Wright, J.; Suen, R.M.; *A Human Clinical Study of Ester-C vs. L-Ascorbic Acid*, Meridian Valley Clinical Laboratory, Kent, Washington, 1988.

59. Kaul, T.N.; et al.; "Antiviral Effect of Flavonoids on Human Viruses," *J. Med. Virol.* 15:71-79, 1985.

60. Werbach, M.; *"Nutritional Influences on Illness,"* Third Line Press, Inc., Tarzana, California, p. 259, 1988.

61. Ames, S.R.; "Factors Affecting Absorption, Transport and Storage of Vitamin A," *Am. J. Clin. Nutr.* 22:934, 1969.

62. Tappel, A.L.; *Nutrition Today*, July-Aug., 1973.

63. Prasad, J.S.; "Effect of Vitamin E on Leukocyte Function," *Am. J. Clin. Nutr.* 33:606-8, 1980.

64. Axelrod, A.E.; Traketellis, A.C.; "Relationship of Pyridoxine to Immunological Phenomena," *Vitam. Horm.* 22:591-607, 1964.

65. Chandra, R.K.; "Nutrition and Immunity—Basic Considerations," Part 1, *Contemp. Nutr.* 11(11), 1986.

66. Levy, J.A.; "Nutrition and the Immune System," in Stites, D.P., et al, *Basic and Clinical Immunology*, fourth edition, Lange Medical Publications, Los Altos, California, pp. 297-305, 1982.

67. Ibid.

68. Beisel, W.R.; Edelman, R.; et al.; "Single Nutrient Effects on Immunologic Function," *J.A.M.A.* 245:53-58, 1981.

69. Das, U.N.; "Antibiotic-Like Action of Essential Fatty Acids," *Can. Med. Assoc. J.* 132:1350, 1985.

70. Bean, W.B.; Hodges, R.E.; Daum, K.; "Pantothenic Acid Deficiency Induced in Human Subjects," *Proc. Soc. Exper. Biol. Med.* 86, pp. 693-698, 1954.

71. Beisel, W.R.; Edelman, R.; et al.; "Single Nutrient Effects on Immunologic Function," *J.A.M.A.* 245:53-58, 1981.

72. Hodges, R.E.; Bean, W.B.; et al.; "Factors Affecting Human Antibody Response," *Am. J. Clin. Nutr.* 11, No. 2, pp. 85-93, 1962.

73. Wara, D.W.; Ammann, A.J.; "Thymosin Treatment of Children with Primary Immunodeficiency Disease," *Transpl. Proc.* 10, No. 1, pp. 203-209, 1978.

74. Bach, J.F.; "Thymic Hormones," *J. Immunophar.* 1, No. 3, pp. 277-310, 1979.

75. Rubenstein, A.; et al.; "In Vivo and In Vitro Effects of Thymosin and Adenosine Deaminase on Adenosine-Deaminase-Deficient Lymphocytes," *New Engl. J. Med.* 300, No. 8, pp. 387-392, 1979.

76. Aiuti, F.; et al.; "Thymopoietin Pentapeptide Treatment of Primary Immunodeficiencies," *Lancet* pp. 551-554, 1983.

77. Paul, S.; "The Virus Crisis," Lecture presented in Bloomington, Minnesota, Feb. 24, 1990.

Index

Dr. Michael A. Schmidt, D.C., C.C.N. is an author, lecturer, and researcher in the field of natural health care. He is a co-author of *Beyond Antibiotics: Healthier Options for Families* and is the author of *Tired of Being Tired: A Guide to Overcoming Fatigue and Low Vitality.* Schmidt is co-author of *Managing the Patient with Chronic Fatigue,* a contributing author to a textbook of family practice and to *The New Medicine,* and the former editor of *Current Topics in Preventive Pediatrics and Family Practice.* Dr. Schmidt was featured as Clinician of the Month on *Preventive Medicine Update* in 1991 and has been a guest on radio and television. His work has appeared in magazines and professional journals.

Dr. Schmidt studied biology and chemistry at Augsburg College, the University of Minnesota, and the University of the State of New York, and was employed in analytical chemistry and microbiology. He received his doctorate from North-western College of Chiropractic in 1982 and is board-certified in clinical nutrition. Dr. Schmidt is on the Scientific Council of the International and American Associations of Clinical Nutritionists, is on the medical advisory board of the FER Foundation for Hearing and Youth, and is on the post-graduate faculty of various institutions. Schmidt's interests in medicine are broad, ranging from nutritional biochemistry to psychoneuroimmunology, but he also emphasizes the art of healing and the role of such things as meaning, compassion, hope, and beliefs. He is invited to lecture internationally on clinical nutrition and preventive medicine, and is pursuing a doctoral degree in behavioral science and molecular biology.

His goal is to build a bridge of understanding between Western allopathic medicine and holistic medicine, presenting the latter in a context that is scientifically respectable. He lives in Anoka, Minnesota with his wife and two sons.